Sleep Medicine in Neurology

NEUROLOGY IN PRACTICE:

SERIES EDITORS:
ROBERT A. GROSS, DEPARTMENT OF NEUROLOGY, UNIVERSITY OF
ROCHESTER MEDICAL CENTER, ROCHESTER, NY, USA

JONATHAN W. MINK, DEPARTMENT OF NEUROLOGY, UNIVERSITY OF
ROCHESTER MEDICAL CENTER, ROCHESTER, NY, USA

Sleep Medicine in Neurology

EDITED BY

Douglas B. Kirsch, MD, FAASM

Harvard Medical School
Boston, MA, USA

and

Division of Sleep Neurology
Department of Neurology
Brigham and Women's Hospital
Boston, MA, USA

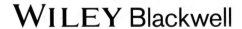

This edition first published 2014 © 2014 by John Wiley & Sons, Ltd

Registered Office
John Wiley & Sons, Ltd, The Atrium, Southern Gate, Chichester, West Sussex, PO19 8SQ, UK

Editorial Offices
9600 Garsington Road, Oxford, OX4 2DQ, UK
The Atrium, Southern Gate, Chichester, West Sussex, PO19 8SQ, UK
111 River Street, Hoboken, NJ 07030–5774, USA

For details of our global editorial offices, for customer services and for information about how to apply for permission to reuse the copyright material in this book please see our website at www.wiley.com/wiley-blackwell.

Library of Congress Cataloging-in-Publication Data

Sleep medicine in neurology / edited by Douglas B Kirsch.
    p. ; cm. – (Neurology in practice)
  Includes bibliographical references and index.
  ISBN 978-1-4443-3551-4 (cloth)
I. Kirsch, Douglas B., editor of compilation.   II. Series: Neurology in practice (Series)
  [DNLM: 1. Sleep Disorders. 2. Nervous System Diseases.   WL 108]
  RC547
  616.8′498–dc23

                          2013023366

A catalogue record for this book is available from the British Library.

Wiley also publishes its books in a variety of electronic formats. Some content that appears in print may not be available in electronic books.

Cover image: ©iStockphoto.com. Inset image courtesy of Dr Douglas B. Kirsch.
Cover design by Sarah Dickinson.

Set in 8.75/11.75pt Utopia by SPi Publisher Services, Pondicherry, India
Printed and bound in Malaysia by Vivar Printing Sdn Bhd

1 2014

Contents

Contributors

Andreea Andrei, MD
Assistant Professor
Menninger Department of Psychiatry
and Behavioral Sciences
Baylor College of Medicine
The Methodist Hospital
Houston
TX, USA

Mihaela H. Bazalakova, MD, PhD
Division of Sleep Medicine
Department of Medicine
Brigham and Women's Hospital
and
Department of Neurology
Massachusetts General Hospital
Boston
MA, USA

Martha E. Billings, MD
Department of Medicine, Division of Pulmonary
Critical Care
University of Washington
UW Medicine Sleep Center
Harborview Medical Center
Seattle
WA, USA

Robert Busch, DMD, MD
Oral and Maxillofacial Surgery Department
The Methodist Hospital Physician Organization
Houston
TX, USA

Melinda Davis-Malessevich, MD
The Bobby R Alford Department of
Otolaryngology – Head and Neck Surgery
Baylor College of Medicine
Houston
TX, USA

Maryann C. Deak, MD
Clinical Instructor, Harvard Medical School
Medical Director, Sleep HealthCenters Beverly
Associate Physician, Brigham and Women's
Hospital
Boston, MA, USA

Lawrence J. Epstein, MD
Division of Sleep Medicine
Department of Medicine
Brigham and Women's Hospital
and
Instructor in Medicine, Harvard Medical School
Boston
MA, USA

Jaime Gateno, DDS, MD
Weill Cornell Medical College
and
Oral and Maxillofacial Surgery Department
The Methodist Hospital
Houston
TX, USA

Aatif M. Husain, MD
Department of Medicine (Neurology)
Duke University Medical Center
and
Neurodiagnostic Center
Veterans Affairs Medical Center
Durham
NC, USA

Makoto Kawai, MD
Department of Neurology
Methodist Neurological Institute
and
Assistant Professor
Weill Cornell Medical College
Houston
TX, USA

Douglas B. Kirsch, MD, FAASM
Harvard Medical School
and
Division of Sleep Neurology
Department of Neurology
Brigham and Women's Hospital
Boston
MA, USA

Ravichand Madala, MD
Department of Neurology
Duke University Medical Center
Durham
NC, USA

Raman Malhotra, MD
SLUCare Sleep Disorders Center
and
Department of Neurology and Psychiatry
Saint Louis University School of Medicine
St Louis
MO, USA

Shalini Paruthi, MD
Saint Louis University School of Medicine
and
Pediatric Sleep and Research Center
SSM Cardinal Glennon Children's Medical Center
St Louis
MO, USA

Rodney A. Radtke, MD
Department of Neurology
Duke University Medical Center
Durham
NC, USA

Mary Rose, PsyD, CBSM
Department of Medicine
Pulmonary, Critical Care and Sleep Medicine
Baylor College of Medicine
Houston
TX, USA

Rajdeep Singh, MD
Department of Neurology,
Carolinas Medical Center
UNC Chapel Hill
Charlotte
NC, USA

Masayoshi Takashima, MD, FACS, FAAOA
Sleep Medicine Fellowship, Otolaryngology –
Head and Neck Surgery Section
The Bobby R Alford Department of
Otolaryngology – Head and Neck Surgery
Baylor College of Medicine
Houston
TX, USA

Sheila C. Tsai, MD
Department of Medicine
National Jewish Health
University of Colorado Denver School
of Medicine
Denver
CO, USA

Nathaniel F. Watson, MD, MSc
Department of Neurology,
University of Washington
UW Medicine Sleep Center
Harborview Medical Center
Seattle
WA, USA

Emerson M. Wickwire, PhD, ABPP, CBSM
Pulmonary Disease and Critical Care Associates
Columbia
MD, USA
and
Department of Psychiatry and Behavioral
Sciences
Johns Hopkins School of Medicine
Baltimore
MD, USA

Scott G. Williams, MD
Department of Pulmonary, Critical Care
and Sleep Medicine
Womack Army Medical Center
Fort Bragg
NC, USA

Series Foreword

The genesis for this book series started with the proposition that, increasingly, physicians want direct, useful information to help them in clinical care. Textbooks, while comprehensive, are useful primarily as detailed reference works but pose challenges for uses at the point of care. By contrast, more outline-type references often leave out the "hows and whys" – pathophysiology, pharmacology – that form the basis of management decisions. Our goal for this series is to present books, covering most areas of neurology, that provide enough background information to allow the reader to feel comfortable, but not so much as to be overwhelming; and to associate that with practical advice from experts about care, combining the growing evidence base with best practices.

Our series will encompass various aspects of neurology, with topics and the specific content chosen to be accessible and useful.

Chapters cover critical information that will inform the reader of the disease processes and mechanisms as a prelude to treatment planning. Algorithms and guidelines are presented, when appropriate. "Tips and Tricks" boxes provide expert suggestions, while other boxes present cautions and warnings to avoid pitfalls. Finally, we provide "Science Revisited" sections that review the most important and relevant science background material, and references and further reading sections that guide the reader to additional material.

We welcome feedback. As additional volumes are added to the series, we hope to refine the content and format so that our readers will be best served.

Our thanks, appreciation, and respect go out to our editors and their contributors, who conceived and refined the content for each volume, assuring a high-quality, practical approach to neurological conditions and their treatment.

Our thanks also go to our mentors and students (past, present, and future), who have challenged and delighted us; to our book editors and their contributors, who were willing to take on additional work for an educational goal; and to our publisher, Martin Sugden, for his ideas and support, for wonderful discussions and commiseration over baseball and soccer teams that might not quite have lived up to expectations. We would like to dedicate the series to Marsha, Jake and Dan; and to Janet, Laura and David. And also to Steven R. Schwid, MD, our friend and colleague, whose ideas helped to shape this project and whose humor brightened our lives, but he could not complete this goal with us.

Robert A. Gross
Jonathan W. Mink
Rochester, NY, USA

Preface

For centuries of scientific exploration, sleep was considered a "black box." Though theories about what happens when humans and animals sleep have been observed in the writings of the ancient Greek philosophers through Rene Descartes and Thomas Willis and into the 19th century, little understanding of the biology of sleep occurred until the 20th century. Over the last 75 years, there has been an explosion of knowledge about the physiological processes in the brain that occur during sleep and the disorders that disrupt normal sleep.

The goal for this book is to review the clinical disorders of sleep for neurologists, but the subject material is likely relevant for a clinical practitioner of any specialty with an interest in sleep medicine. In today's medical community, assessment of sleeping problems continues to be a mystery for many clinicians, mostly related to a dearth of sleep-related education in medical school and training programs. However, much information is now available about the links between sleep disorders and other medical conditions, including factors relevant to many clinicians' daily practice. For instance, as neurologists consider modifiable risk factors for stroke prevention, methods of helping patients minimize headache frequency, and improving quality of life for patients with dementia, they should be considering disorders of sleep and how to address them. Hopefully, upon reviewing the chapters of this text, the reader will feel more comfortable conversing with their patients about sleep disorders and discussing possible treatment options.

Certification for sleep medicine in the United States requires a year-long fellowship after completing one of several residency programs, including neurology, internal medicine, psychiatry, and pediatrics. We are unable to replicate that learning process in this (or any) book. However, our hope is that this text provides a readable, clinically relevant source of information about sleep and its disorders, useful for any stage of medical practice from resident to attending physician. Particular tips, tricks, and cautions are highlighted in boxes throughout each chapter to increase the reader's yield. This book introduces the topic of sleep medicine in the first chapter, discussing some of the background history and growth of the field. The second and third chapters review the clinical approach to the patient with a sleep problem and the possible options for subjective and objective testing. The following chapters describe in detail each of the major sleep disorders, including insomnia, parasomnias, hypersomnia, sleep-disordered breathing, and limb symptoms. In addition, there are chapters devoted to the specific relationships between sleep and neurological disorders and the effects of sleep disorders on cognition and driving. The final chapter reviews aspects of pediatric sleep medicine, particularly highlighting those that differ from their adult counterparts.

As a neurologist who didn't even know sleep medicine was a subspecialty of neurology until late in my residency, I can only hope that the readers of this book, from whatever specialty, end up finding sleep medicine as exciting as I do.

Douglas B. Kirsch, MD
Boston, MA

Acknowledgments

Thanks go:

To Julie Elliott, from Oxford for keeping us all running like Swiss clocks … on time.
To Drs. Gross and Mink, for resuscitating a project nearing asystole.
To My parents, who let me choose my own adventure, while providing guidance along the way.
To Ryan, who smiles at me when I wake him up in the morning and when I put him to bed at night.
And to Erin, who supports what I do and amazingly enough loves me for who I am.

Introduction to Sleep Medicine

Douglas B. Kirsch, MD, FAASM

Harvard Medical School and Division of Sleep Neurology, Department of Neurology, Brigham and Women's Hospital, USA

Introduction

Sleep medicine is a field which has had exponential growth over the last 25 years. Interest has blossomed from both medical practitioners and the general public on the impact sleep has on human function and long-term health. Sleep clinics and laboratories have become more common and an enlarging market of consumer goods for home analysis of sleep has developed. This chapter will introduce you to the field of sleep medicine, describe normal sleep, and provide a basic outline of the sleep disorders.

The American Medical Association recognized sleep medicine as a specialty in 1995. The field of sleep medicine is currently composed of physicians from many specialties. In fact, physicians from six American Board of Medical Specialties (ABMS) primary boards are able to sit for the board examination in sleep medicine: the American Boards of Psychiatry and Neurology, Internal Medicine, Pediatrics, Anesthesiology, Family Medicine, and Otolaryngology. This blend of primary specialties leads to a vibrant subspecialty with a variety of interests ranging from airway anatomy to snoring surveys.

> ⚡ CAUTION
>
> As of 2013, to qualify to sit for the ABMS examination, an Accreditation Council for Graduate Medical Education (ACGME)-certified Sleep Medicine Fellowship must be completed. Before 2013, entry could be obtained via a practice-based experimental pathway.

A brief history of sleep and sleep medicine

Sleep has been of interest to cultures for thousands of years. Ancient Egyptians devoted sections of papyri to the interpretation of dreaming. In the ancient Greek culture, Aristotle wrote a work entitled *On Sleep and Sleeplessness* devoted to sleep and waking; he also believed that ingesting food caused sleepiness through "fumes" that were carried through the blood vessels into the brain. Hippocrates, considered by some to be the father of Greek medicine, wrote this about sleep and its relationship to health.[1]

> 'With regard to sleep – as is usual with us in health, the patient should wake during the day and sleep during the night. If this rule be anywise altered it is so far worse: but there will be little harm provided he sleep in the morning for the third part of the day; such sleep as takes place after this time is more unfavorable; but the worst of all is to get no sleep either night or day; for it follows from this symptom that the insomnolency is connected with sorrow and pains, or that he is about to become delirious.'

The Bible discusses the prophecies that occurred through dreaming, most notable in the story of Joseph. A religious text from the Judaic faith, written by a scholar known as Maimonides in the 1100s, stated the following, which still holds true today.[2]

> 'The day and night consist of 24 hours. It is sufficient for a person to sleep one-third thereof which is eight hours. These should be at the end

of the night so that from the beginning of sleep until the rising of the sun will be eight hours. Thus he will arise from his bed before the sun rises.'

It is not until the 17th century that medical theories around sleep clearly resurface after the long Dark Ages. Rene Descartes developed a hydraulic model of sleep, involving movement of the pituitary gland. Thomas Willis described patients with symptoms of narcolepsy and restless legs syndrome. The science of circadian rhythms was brought to light in the mid-18th century by Jean Jacques d'Ortous de Mairan, when he described that a heliotrope plant kept a stable pattern of opening its blooms for the day, even when kept in a dark environment without the sun for a cue.

Multiple theories about sleep circulated in the 19th century: sleep was related to changes in blood flow, sleep was caused by an increase in toxins in the blood, or sleep was initiated by physical changes in the newly discovered neurons. Increasing research was done on the changes in temperature in the human body. William Hammond, a physician during the Civil War, wrote *Sleep and Its Derangements* in 1869, primarily discussing insomnia; likely the first text on the subject in the Americas.

In 1925, Hans Berger measured the electrical activity of the human brain, via his "Elektrenkephalogramm". Two groups, one at Harvard University and one at the University of Chicago, used this device to perform the majority of sleep-related research in the late 1930s. Alfred Loomis's group at Harvard categorized sleep into stages A to E, from the electrical brain rhythm of wakefulness to stages of deep non-rapid eye movement (NREM) sleep, in order of resistance to change by disturbance. Nathaniel Kleitman and his student Eugene Aserinsky discovered rapid eye movement (REM) sleep in 1953 at the University of Chicago after observation of episodic eye movements during sleep in infants. They developed the electrooculogram (EOG) to better characterize the eye movements, noting both rapid and slow eye motions. Kleitman and William Dement then applied these studies to demonstrate the recurring pattern of REM and NREM sleep; sleep was no longer a purely homogenous state with low-frequency electroencephalogram (EEG) readings, much to the surprise of many others working in the field.

In 1967, Allan Rechtschaffen and Anthony Kales, as well as others, developed a scoring manual for human sleep. A *Manual of Standardized Terminology, Techniques, and Scoring System for Sleep Stages of Human Subjects* was published in 1968 with the hope that it would "markedly increase the comparability of results reported by different investigators." This monograph formally defined the polysomnogram and clarifying the stages of sleep (wakefulness, movement time, stages 1–4 [NREM sleep], and REM sleep). The Multiple Sleep Latency Test was developed at Stanford in the early 1980s to evaluate narcoleptics and their daytime sleep propensity. In 2008, the scoring manual for sleep was reviewed, updated and renamed (*AASM Manual for the Scoring of Sleep and Associated Events: Rules, Terminology and Technical Specifications*); another update was undertaken in 2012.

The modern clinic for evaluating and treating patients with sleep disorders was developed at Stanford University in its Sleep Disorders Clinic which had initially began in the 1960s, closed, and then re-opened in 1970. Other sleep clinics began to spread across the United States, eventually grouping together to form the American Academy of Sleep Medicine. The number of sleep laboratories or centers has grown steadily since the mid-1990s and today there are an estimated 3000–3500 sleep laboratories operating in the United States.

Normal sleep

Thomas Edison once said: "In my opinion sleep is a habit, acquired by the environment. Like all habits, it is generally carried to extremes. The man that sleeps four hours soundly is better off than the dreamy sleeper of eight hours."[3] However, recent data have demonstrated that not only is 8 hours of sleep not a detriment for most people, it is a necessary component for optimal functioning. People who obtain insufficient sleep are prone to difficulties with attention, may suffer from cognitive and mood problems, and appear to be at higher risk for co-morbid medical disorders and death, particularly in those with less than 6 hours of sleep per night. However, epidemiological studies of sleep times suggest not only that people with inadequate sleep times are more likely to die sooner, but that people with excessive sleep times (more than 9 hours per night) are also at increased risk, potentially due to underlying illness.[4]

In the general population, excessive daytime sleepiness is most commonly caused by insufficient nighttime sleep rather than a primary sleep disorder. Adequate sleep is often traded for work or social activities. A brief review of the patient's sleep schedule may be helpful.

Sleep changes over the course of our lives. Newborn babies spend about 50% of their total sleep in REM sleep, and in fact enter sleep via REM sleep, which is not considered normal in adults. Newborns also sleep in short episodes initially (as any new parent is aware), though they may obtain 12–18 hours of sleep over the course of the day. During the first few months of life, infants consolidate sleep into longer blocks which occur at night, attempting to acquire 14–15 hours of sleep per day. As children reach school age (5–10 years old), their daily sleep demand decreases to 10–11 hours. Teenagers require 8.5–9.25 hours of sleep per night (often getting less than that due to school commitments and social interests), and adults need 7–9 hours. In rare confirmed cases, it appears that humans with certain genetics are "short sleepers" and require less sleep than the average. Much more commonly, modern adults obtain less sleep than they require to perform optimally, distracted by long work schedules or the wealth of available entertainment options. Later in life, older adults generally require similar amounts of sleep (7–9 hours), though it becomes more difficult for them to maintain sleep consolidation with medical disorders and medications and napping may become more common.

While many people expect older adults to require less sleep than young adults, sleep requirements are not dramatically different. Clinical attention should be paid to napping schedules, circadian pattern, and possible underlying sleep and medical disorders.

The clear purpose of sleep is not truly known, though each of us is acutely aware of its regenerative properties for alertness. However, many other functions appear to occur during the night, most prominently memory processing, hormonal fluctuation, and metabolic changes. While one theory suggests that sleep allows an organism to save energy, functional brain scans during sleep reveal that the human brain is more active in some areas during REM sleep than when awake, and the energy savings appear to be about the number of calories in one cookie. The high neuronal activity observed in REM sleep may be part of the education process, strengthening and weakening synapses related to things we learned (or didn't learn) during the period of wakefulness preceding sleep. Alternatively, or perhaps adjunctively, memory extraction and filing may represent the notable magnetic resonance imaging (MRI) signal activity. The immune system appears positively affected by sleep; animal species that sleep longer appear to have fewer parasites and higher white blood cell counts.

Almost all living creatures have a circadian clock, so that certain functions of the organism occur at optimal times. As pointed out in the historical section, even the simple heliotrope flower has an internal clock, so that it might bloom at the optimal time each day (even if the sun is not present). Humans have a similar clock, such that our tendency is generally to sleep when it is dark outside and be awake during the sunlit portion of the day. Some mammals, such as mice, have a reversed clock, in which they have a tendency to be awake in the nocturnal portion of the cycle. Our circadian cycle is relevant from a physiological perspective, in that many hormones (growth hormone, melatonin, cortisol) appear at different times during our 24-hours cycle. However, our clock also affects how we respond to plane travel (jet-lag) and working non-standard shifts (night work, rotating shifts). Our sleep patterns in relationship to this clock also have a tendency to shift as we age, such that teenagers biologically tend to have a delayed sleep phase and older adults tend to have an advanced sleep phase.

An easy way to remember the shift of the circadian sleep phase over the lifespan is to consider teenagers; they never want to get up in the morning to go to school, but are always ready to stay up late at night to watch TV or play video games. Meanwhile, in Florida, you might find your grandmother walking the beach before the sun rises in the morning, but dozing off in her chair while watching TV in the early evening.

Currently, the clinical evaluation of sleep is performed most commonly by an in-laboratory polysomnogram (sleep study) (Figure 1.1). Via measurement of brain waves (EEG), eye movements (EOG), heart rate and rhythm (electrocardiography, EKG), muscle movement of chin and legs (electromyography, EMG), nasal pressure and airflow (nasal-oral thermistor), chest and thorax movement, and oximetry, these studies allow for assessment of sleep stage, breathing, and movements during sleep. Video monitoring is standard to allow for assessment of parasomnias and other behaviors. A polysomnographic technologist

places the leads on the patient, monitors them through the night, and unhooks them in the morning.

The overnight test typically runs overnight for a minimum of 6 hours, but often longer. These studies are visually scored in 30-sec increments. The current scoring manual categorizes sleep into several stages: wake, N1, N2, N3, and R. Stages N1–N3 are progressively deeper stages of what is considered NREM sleep. N1 is considered light sleep, usually what occurs when a person transitions from wake into sleep. The majority of NREM sleep during the night in a normal individual is stage N2. Stage N3, also known as slow-wave sleep, appears most frequently in children and young adults, lessening in frequency as we age. Stage R, also known as REM sleep, is a time of skeletal muscle atonia (except eye and breathing muscles) which is strongly associated with vivid dreaming. The breathing and heart rhythm in stage R tend to be more irregular in pattern. The majority of sleep (perhaps 75–80%) in a normal adult is spent in NREM sleep; episodes of

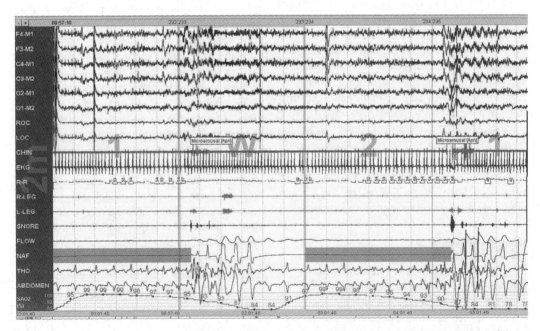

Figure 1.1 Two-minute epoch of in-laboratory polysomnography (Nihon Khoden, Foothill Ranch, CA) from a 55-year-old man with obstructive sleep apnea. The top six leads are EEG (right and left frontal, central, and occipital), followed by two eye leads (right and left), the chin lead, ECG with heart rate below (R-R), two leg leads (right and left), snore channel, oronasal thermistor, nasal pressure transducer, effort bands (thorax and abdomen), and oxygen saturation. Two obstructive apneas are observed at the boxes in the NAF (nasal airflow) signal with absent nasal-oral airflow and continued respiratory effort. The respiratory events are associated with increased frequency signal (arousals) in the EEG signals and oxygen desaturations.

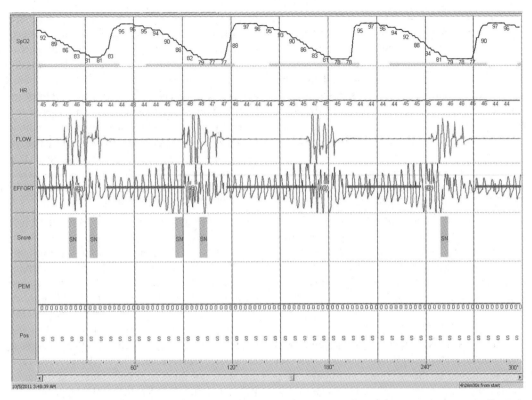

Figure 1.2 This is a 5-minute epoch from a Stardust home sleep testing device (Respironics, Murrysville, PA) of a 64-year-old woman with obstructive sleep apnea. The top channel is oximetry, followed by heart rate, nasal pressure, respiratory effort, snoring, patient event marker (PEM), and position (in this case, supine). The epoch demonstrates repetitive apneas with absent nasal pressure and continuous respiratory effort.

REM sleep occur every 90–120 min and account for approximately 20–25% of the total sleep time.

In some cases, daytime studies are performed to evaluate the presence of daytime sleepiness or to assess the ability to maintain alertness (the Multiple Sleep Latency Test and the Maintenance of Wakefulness Test respectively). These will be covered more fully in the chapter on assessment of excessive daytime sleepiness. More recently, testing for obstructive sleep apnea has been done in the home rather than the laboratory (Figure 1.2); this home testing is undertaken via assessment of breathing, but most home monitors do not include an actual evaluation of sleep.

Sleep disorders: a brief review

There are many ways to categorize sleep disorders. One is the *International Classification of Sleep Disorders*, currently in its second edition (ICSD-2). Box 1.1 lists the broad categories it uses.

> **Box 1.1 ICSD-2 sleep disorder categories**
>
> Insomnia
>
> Sleep-related breathing disorders
>
> Hypersomnias of central origin
>
> Circadian rhythm sleep disorder
>
> Parasomnias
>
> Sleep-related movement disorders
>
> Isolated symptoms, apparently normal variants, and unresolved issues
>
> Other sleep disorders

An alternative method of categorization is to consolidate disorders into broader groups: disorders of sleep fragmentation (insomnia, sleep-disordered breathing), disorders of wake (hypersomnias, circadian rhythms), and abnormal activities during sleep (sleep-related movement disorders and parasomnias). Whether you lump or split these disorders, it is important to understand how to appropriately assess and treat your patients. This section will briefly discuss the disorders, each of which will be reviewed in more detail in the chapters to follow.

Insomnias

This group of disorders is defined by difficulty falling asleep, staying asleep, waking too early, or feeling unrefreshed in the morning, usually associated with some form of daytime impact. A nearly universal experience which may be related to stress, medical conditions, or medications, insomnia is generally time-limited, lasting only a few days or weeks. However, in approximately 10% of the United States population, the disorder is chronic.

Sleep-related breathing disorders

Obstructive sleep apnea, central sleep apnea, and hypoventilation are the primary disorders relevant to neurologists in this section. Obstructive sleep apnea, the most common disorder diagnosed in sleep laboratories, is caused by collapse of the upper airway, resulting in arousals and daytime sleepiness. Particularly relevant is that patients with obstructive apnea are at increased risk for hypertension, coronary artery disease, and strokes. Central sleep apnea occurs when breathing stops with an open airway due to a disorder in the respiratory control circuit. While it most commonly occurs in patients with congestive heart failure, it may also arise transiently or permanently in patients after strokes or with other brain diseases. Hypoventilation, where gas exchange is insufficient to rid the body of carbon dioxide and bring in enough oxygen, appears in patients who suffer from certain cardiopulmonary disorders, obesity, or neuromuscular conditions, such as amyotrophic lateral sclerosis.

Hypersomnias

The hypersomnias, particularly narcolepsy, are a common reason for referral to a sleep center, but are rarely the diagnosed disorder. Generally speaking, narcolepsy and idiopathic hypersomnia are fairly rare disorders resulting in significant daytime sleepiness causing impairment in function. The pentad of narcoleptic symptoms includes hypersomnia, sleep paralysis, hypnogogic hallucinations, cataplexy, and insomnia (almost always in the form of sleep fragmentation). While not all patients with narcolepsy have cataplexy, when it occurs, it is typically pathognomic for the disorder. Idiopathic hypersomnia appears to have a different pathophysiology from narcolepsy and appears in two forms in the current ICSD-2, with long sleep time and without long sleep time, depending on whether the length of time of the primary nocturnal sleep is more or less than 10 hours.

Circadian rhythm sleep disorder

As mentioned previously, humans have a circadian clock that dictates their preferred sleeping hours. However, when that preferred sleep time does not match with their expected schedule, a sleeping problem is likely to occur. These mismatches present in patients flying across several time zones (jet-lag), with work shifts that start very early in the morning, are overnight, or which rotate over the course of the week (shift work), or perhaps most commonly, when patients have a daytime schedule that does not meet with their biological desire to stay up late and sleep late (delayed sleep phase).

Parasomnias

Confusional arousals, sleepwalking, sleep-related eating disorder, and enuresis (bedwetting) are some of the more common abnormal sleep-related behaviors, classified as parasomnias. Children are more prone to these disorders than adults in general. In specific parasomnias, such as REM-sleep behavior disorder, when patients enact dream-related behavior at a typical time of atonia, adults are the more common demographic, particularly those with underlying alpha-synucleinopathies.

Sleep-related movement disorders

Sleep-related movement disorders include diagnoses such as restless legs syndrome (RLS), periodic limb movement disorder, and sleep-related bruxism (teeth grinding). They are typically characterized by simple stereotyped movements that disrupt sleep, though RLS is a more complex set of movements and was lumped in this group due to its association with periodic limb movements. Patients with RLS very commonly have periodic limb movements on their polysomnograms (about 80%), though only a small portion of patients with periodic limb movements on polysomnograms (about 20%) have RLS. Sleep-related bruxism is most common in children and occurs in about 8% of adults.

Isolated symptoms

This group is an assortment of unrelated diagnoses, including snoring, myoclonic jerks (sleep starts), and long and short sleepers. According to some reports, snoring occurs in 24% of adult women and 40% of adult men. However, there is ongoing debate as to whether snoring, in the absence of obstructive sleep apnea, is associated with morbidity. Myoclonic jerks which occur on the transition from wake to sleep are very common, generally benign, and are often only observed by the bed partner (unless, of course, you are falling asleep in a public place).

Other sleep disorders

Lastly, the "Other sleep disorders" include those cases in which it is unclear what the final sleep disorder will be or when diagnoses appear to overlap. The most clear disorder in this category is environmental sleep disorder, in which a "physically measurable stimulus" causes disruption of sleep and a resultant fragmentation of sleep or daytime sleepiness.

Helpful resources

While the hope is that this book will provide an in-depth review of important topics in sleep medicine, there are other resources that may expand the reader's knowledge on a specific topic or be useful in the care of patients with sleep disorders.

- *American Academy of Sleep Medicine*: the AASM is "the only professional society dedicated exclusively to the medical subspecialty of sleep medicine." This group has produced many practice parameters for sleep medicine as well as a standardized scoring manual for sleep: www.aasmnet. org. The AASM also provides some useful information for patients at: http://yoursleep. aasmnet.org/.
- *American Thoracic Society*: this professional society, composed of many specialties including pulmonary and critical care physicians dedicated to the chest and lungs, provides good educational materials regarding sleep: www. thoracic.org/clinical/sleep/index.php.

- *Centers for Disease Control*: the US government has a website providing education on sleep topics, including insufficient sleep and sleep disorders: www.cdc.gov/sleep/.
- *National Sleep Foundation*: this organization is "dedicated to improving sleep health and safety through education, public awareness, and advocacy." It has resources for both physicians and patients on its website: www.sleepfoundation.org.

The future of sleep medicine

Sleep medicine has been a growing specialty in the last few decades with increasing interest from scientific researchers and the public. Demand from patients for consultation on sleeping problems is likely to continue to climb in the United States, in both adult and child populations. Changes are likely to occur in assessment and treatment modalities, with an increasing shift from the sleep laboratory towards home-based diagnosis and management. Sleep medicine physicians will need to implement long-term follow-up plans for patients with chronic disorders, such as those with insomnia or obstructive sleep apnea, similar to treatment for diabetes or hypertension.

References

1. Hippocrates. *The Book of Prognostics* (part 10). Digital Hippocrates website: www.chlt.org/sandbox/dh/Adams/page.49.a.php (accessed June 2013).
2. Rosner F. The hygienic principles of Moses Maimonides. *JAMA* 1965; **194**(13): 1352–4 .
3. Pollak C, Thorpy M, Yager J. *The Encyclopedia of Sleep and Sleep Disorders*, 2nd edn. New York: Facts on File, 2001.
4. Cappuccio FP, D'Elia L, Strazzullo P. Sleep duration and all-cause mortality: a systematic review and meta-analysis of prospective studies. *Sleep* 2010; **33**(5): 585–92.

Further reading

American Academy of Sleep Medicine. *International Classification of Sleep Disorders*, 2nd edn. Westchester, IL: American Academy of Sleep Medicine, 2005.

Kirsch DB. There and back again: a current history of sleep medicine. *Chest* 2011; **139**(4): 939–46.

2

The History and Physical Examination of the Sleep Patient

Sheila C. Tsai, MD

Department of Medicine, National Jewish Health, University of Colorado Denver, USA

Introduction

Sleep disorders affect millions of people in the United States and worldwide. As the importance of sleep on health is increasingly recognized, more patients are presenting with sleep issues. It is important to have the necessary tools and skills to assess these problems. In this chapter, important aspects of the history and physical examination that can help pinpoint the diagnosis are discussed. We also review helpful points to consider when evaluating patients in order to avoid making common mistakes.

A number of sleep disorders exist; the categories range from disorders of sleepiness, or hypersomnia, to disorders resulting in insomnia. Also included are circadian rhythm abnormalities and sleep-related breathing disorders. Given the breadth of the disorders associated with sleep, the sleep history is necessarily extensive and detailed. As with all medical practice, a good history allows the clinician to use targeted questions to determine an etiology for patient symptoms. Key physical examination elements aid the evaluation and help support specific diagnoses.

The sleep history

A sleep disorder can often be diagnosed by history alone. For example, restless legs syndrome is a diagnosis based on clinical presentation and symptoms that does not need further testing to confirm its presence. Patients have certain key symptoms (criteria) that are met to warrant this diagnosis.

Some common disorders such as insomnia are also defined by the clinical complaints. In obtaining the sleep history, one should start by determining the presenting symptom or primary reason the patient has come for evaluation. Certain questions should be asked of all or most patients, but the history should be honed based on the presenting complaints.

General sleep questions

The chief complaint should be elicited. The patient's thoughts regarding the sleep issue and how it affects daytime functioning or quality of life should be obtained. Patients should be queried on the duration of symptoms, alleviating and exacerbating factors, and a possible trigger to the onset of the problem. Key elements also include a patient's sleep habits and sleep schedule. It is important to determine the sleep schedule on weekdays, weekends, work nights, school nights, and vacation. Knowing this schedule helps discern circadian abnormalities or the influence of work hours on sleep duration and timing. Questions about unintentional and intentional napping can be helpful. While taking the sleep schedule history, one should ask the length of time it takes to fall asleep and whether there are difficulties staying asleep once the patient has fallen asleep. These questions will help assess insomnia complaints. If sleep quality is poor, attempting to determine an etiology for the disrupted sleep is beneficial. For example, the

Sleep Medicine in Neurology, First Edition. Edited by Douglas B. Kirsch.
© 2014 John Wiley & Sons, Ltd. Published 2014 by John Wiley & Sons, Ltd.

presence of abnormal events at night that disrupt sleep should be determined.

Information from a bed partner or family member can be particularly helpful with regard to abnormal events at night. Sometimes, these other household members have prompted the initial evaluation due to concerns about the patient or the effects of the sleep issues on others in the house. They can discuss the specific circumstances surrounding an event during sleep, such as the behaviors and timing of the events. They can attest to abnormal sleep schedules, inadequate sleep hygiene, snoring, pauses in breathing, dream enactment, and other nocturnal events. They can also comment on daytime symptoms such as frequent, unintentional dozing.

It is also important to consider the sleep complaints in the context of the patient's age, gender, and duration of symptoms when evaluating the patient. Certain disorders are more common at different stages in life and therefore, if appropriate, questions should be directed to assess for these disorders.

> ★ **TIPS AND TRICKS**
>
> It is important to consider the history in the context of the patient's age, sex, and underlying medical conditions. The sleep disorders tend to have a sex and age preference and may be more closely associated with certain medical conditions.

Focusing the history

Beyond the general elements of a sleep history, the interview should center around the chief complaints with questions geared towards determining the underlying etiology. The majority of sleep complaints can be divided into excessive sleepiness, difficulties with falling asleep or staying asleep, and abnormal behaviors or sensations associated with sleep. Dividing the sleep disorders into broad categories can help guide the patient interview and focus the assessment of the patient. Recognizing the common sleep disorders that fall into the broad sleep categories (see Table 2.1) also helps direct the evaluation. For example, in a patient with sleepiness, it will be important to ask about cataplexy and snoring to differentiate narcolepsy and sleep-disordered breathing.

Table 2.1 Major sleep-related symptoms and associated disorders

Symptom	Associated sleep disorder
Sleepiness (may manifest as hyperactivity in children)	Chronic insufficient sleep
	Circadian rhythm sleep disorder
	Delayed sleep phase syndrome
	Advanced sleep phase syndrome
	Shift work sleep disorder
	Jet-lag disorder
	Poor sleep hygiene
	Behaviorally induced insufficient sleep syndrome
	Recurrent hypersomnia
	Menstruation-related recurrent hypersomnia
	Klein–Levin syndrome
	Sleep-disordered breathing:
	Obstructive sleep apnea syndrome
	Central sleep apnea syndrome
	Upper airways resistance syndrome
	Medication related
	Substance use/abuse
	Co-morbid with other underlying medical conditions
	Disorders of primary hypersomnia
	Narcolepsy
	Idiopathic hypersomnia
	Traumatic brain injury
	Restless legs syndrome/periodic limb movement disorder
Insomnia	Primary insomnia
	Psychophysiological insomnia
	Paradoxical insomnia
	Co-morbid insomnia
	Circadian rhythm sleep disorder
	Sleep-disordered breathing
	Medication related
	Substance use/abuse
	Restless legs syndrome/periodic limb movement disorder
Abnormal nocturnal events	Confusional arousal
	Night terror
	Sleepwalking/talking/eating
	Rapid eye movement sleep behavior disorder
	Nightmare disorder
	Restless legs syndrome/periodic limb movement disorder
	Sleep paralysis
	Sleep hallucinations

⚠ CAUTION

A specific sleep disorder should not be diagnosed solely on a single complaint in the absence of a comprehensive evaluation. Without a full picture, one may incorrectly diagnose and treat a patient for insomnia. However, if a more thorough history were obtained, concurrent complaints of daytime sleepiness and napping could suggest poor sleep hygiene, obstructive sleep apnea, or a circadian rhythm abnormality.

Sleepiness

A number of factors may contribute to sleepiness but following a systematic interview approach can elicit the underlying factors.

The sleep schedule

Information regarding the sleep schedule is of paramount importance. Knowing the sleep schedule allows one to determine if the patient is getting enough sleep during their major sleep period. Chronically obtaining an insufficient amount of sleep is one of the most common causes for daytime sleepiness and is often underrecognized. A bedtime and wake time shifted either significantly later or earlier than conventional bedtimes can suggest an underlying circadian rhythm abnormality that is contributing to sleepiness. A varied sleep schedule could support the diagnosis of shift work sleep disorder in those working rotating or night shifts. The lack of a single, prolonged sleep period over a 24-hours period supports other possible circadian rhythm abnormalities such as irregular sleep-wake circadian rhythm sleep disorder as well as a potential underlying psychiatric disorder. A sleep schedule that is different on work days, non-work days, school days, non-school days, and vacation can also lead one to suspect these above-mentioned etiologies for sleepiness.

Poor sleep hygiene may also contribute to or perpetuate an unconventional sleep schedule and therefore understanding a patient's sleep habits is important. Electronics use (e.g. television, video games, computer) and behavioral factors can lead to a delay in bedtime. Furthermore, sleep habits and sleep schedule can implicate other co-morbid diseases. For example, spending prolonged amounts of time in bed could be a sign of depression.

Age, presentation, and duration of the symptoms

In children, snoring suggests obstructive sleep apnea syndrome, which peaks between the ages of 2 and 8 years in children when the tonsils are at their largest comparative to the size of the airway. Children may not display sleepiness as a symptom but instead are likely to have hyperactivity or attention difficulty, which may mimic symptoms of attention deficit hyperactivity disorder.

Sleepiness that presents in adolescence or young adulthood suggests delayed sleep phase syndrome and should raise questions regarding primary sleep drive disorders such as narcolepsy. Behaviorally induced insufficient sleep syndrome is common in this age group as social and academic demands increase. Poor sleep hygiene and behavioral issues may also perpetuate sleep problems. Substance use tends to begin in adolescents and young adults as well; thus, exploring substance use and abuse is crucial. Sleepiness that occurs in a cyclical or recurrent pattern may indicate a circadian rhythm abnormality or less commonly, a menstruation-related hypersomnia or Klein–Levin syndrome. Therefore, questions should aim to evaluate these disorders. Questions regarding recurrent hypersomnias should assess whether there is a monthly association of hypersomnia with the menstrual cycle or if there is associated hypersexuality or hyperphagia, as would be seen in Klein–Levin syndrome.

Sleepiness presenting in middle-aged adults may be more likely to occur from sleep-disordered breathing or circadian rhythm abnormalities such as shift work disorder. In women, sleep apnea incidence increases after menopause, possibly due to loss of the protective effect of estrogen. The timing of sleepiness during the day can be helpful: morning sleepiness may suggest a delayed sleep phase disorder and early evening sleepiness could be caused by an advanced sleep phase disorder. Sleepiness occurring during night shifts suggests shift work sleep disorder.

Furthermore, co-morbid medical conditions and medication use increase with advancing age so medications should be explored as contributors to sleepiness. Meanwhile, other medical conditions that may manifest with sleepiness should be considered. For example, the risk of stroke and dementia increases with advancing age. These neurological disorders can worsen sleep-disordered breathing, circadian rhythm abnormalities, insomnia, and parasomnias.

Sleep continuity

Sleep continuity should be reviewed with the patient. If sleep is fragmented with nocturnal arousals, one should delve into the cause. Sleep-disordered breathing can lead to fitful sleep and therefore, patients and their bed partners should be questioned regarding loud, disruptive snoring, witnessed pauses in breathing, snore or snort arousals, and gasp awakenings. Worsening of snoring frequency or volume or increased apneas in the supine position are a common finding in obstructive sleep apnea. Nocturia, anxiety, and hot flashes could also be major contributors to sleep fragmentation and serve as clues to other underlying medical conditions.

Naps

Whether a patient takes intentional naps or falls asleep unintentionally can help gauge the severity of daytime sleepiness. The duration and timing of naps should be explored. For example, short, refreshing, and nearly irresistable naps are often noted in narcolepsy, whereas in idiopathic hypersomnia and sleep apnea syndromes, the naps can often be longer and unrefreshing. The timing of naps will often affect the patient's ability to fall asleep at night or perpetuate a circadian rhythm abnormality such as delayed sleep phase syndrome. Importantly, sleepiness and unintentional dozing episodes should be evaluated in the context of safety for the patient and for the public, particularly for those patients in the transportation industry or in safety monitoring positions.

Primary disorders of sleepiness

Primary hypersomnias should be considered when no sleep disruptor or other sleep disorder contributing to sleepiness is elicited. Other causes of sleepiness such as traumatic brain injury, medications, substance use, and other sleep disruptors should be ruled out.

Specific questions are helpful in the evaluation. The tetrad of narcolepsy symptoms includes hypersomnia, cataplexy, hypnogogic/hypnopompic hallucinations, and sleep paralysis, and each should be assessed. The presence of cataplexy is pathognomonic for narcolepsy, but one should avoid influencing a patient's responses. One may ask if the patient notes any unusual occurrences during episodes of intense emotions, such as extreme laughter, anger, or stress. The muscle groups most commonly affected by cataplexy are the knees and jaw. The associated hallucinations occur on the edges of sleep and most commonly are visual but may also be auditory. Sleep paralysis occurs most commonly upon waking from sleep and while it is associated with narcolepsy, it may also be an idiopathic finding of little concern. Patients with narcolepsy also may complain of difficulty maintaining sleep at night. Determining the amount of sleep a patient needs to feel refreshed is also helpful. Patients who are long sleepers may require upwards of 10 hours of sleep to feel alert during the day.

Insomnia

Insomnia is one of the most common symptoms presenting to a primary care provider. Knowing the duration of symptoms helps determine the acuity of the problem and the propensity to experience these sleep issues.

In childhood, behavioral sleep issues such as limit-setting sleep disorder or sleep-onset association disorder can be perceived as insomnia by the caregiver. In limit-setting sleep disorder, the child stalls or refuses to go to bed, requiring significant effort on the part of the caregiver to get the child to sleep. In sleep-onset association disorder, circumstances or objects, such as a blanket, are needed in order to achieve sleep. Anxiety or stress may also cause difficulties with sleep. Furthermore, the onset of idiopathic insomnia usually begins in childhood.

Eliciting a trigger to the episodes of insomnia is helpful. Primary idiopathic insomnia, which is fairly uncommon, tends to be long standing and has been present since childhood without a clear precipitant. Often stress or hormonal issues may contribute to insomnia, and it is important to evaluate whether one of those precipitating factors is present. If insomnia was associated with a primary stressor but persists despite resolution of that stressor, this is often suggestive of psychophysiological insomnia. In this disorder, anxiety is associated with the sleep issue and insomnia tends to improve when the person sleeps in a different environment such as on vacation. Often the negative thoughts surrounding sleep and its impact on quality of life perpetuate the difficulty in sleeping.

Explore how patients perceive their insomnia, their level of debilitation, and the consequences of their poor sleep. Determine how the insomnia affects daytime functioning such as causing chronic fatigue, difficulty concentrating, or irritabilitiy. Insomniacs generally complain of fatigue or tiredness but when specifically queried about true daytime sleepiness, this symptom is frequently not present.

For insomniacs, it is vital to explore previously trialed therapies and their successes or reasons for failure. It is also helpful to assess alleviating and exacerbating factors for the insomnia. One should inquire about sleep aids, both prescription and over the counter, as well as other supplements or herbs that have been tried. Patients have often self-medicated prior to seeking medical assistance, and not infrequently, over-the-counter medications, family members' or friends' prescription medications, and substances such as alcohol have been used to varying degrees and have resulted in different levels of efficacy. Exploring what has been tried in the past also influences what therapies may be suggested, as does the patient's perspective of what might be effective for him or her. That being said, it is worthwhile for the practitioner to remember that previously ineffective medications may still be useful in the correct situation.

It is important to identify contributing conditions to assist in insomnia management. Treating underlying medical conditions can be helpful. For example, treating anxiety or hormonal issues may help with insomnia management. If sleep is fragmented, trying to identify a potential cause is important. Some patients with sleep apnea syndromes may actually present with insomnia as a complaint rather than sleepiness, and therefore, screening for sleep apnea should be undertaken. It is also important to investigate co-existing sleep complaints. The concurrent complaints of insomnia and excessive daytime sleepiness often suggests a circadian rhythm abnormality. However, it could also point to a sleep disorder such as periodic limb movement disorder, in which nocturnal sleep is disrupted leading both to insomnia complaints and to daytime sleepiness.

The sleep schedule

As with assessment of sleepiness, determining the sleep schedule is fundamental. Often, circadian rhythm sleep disorders may masquerade as insomnia. For example, delayed sleep phase syndrome patients may complain of difficulty falling asleep at night, particularly if their natural time to fall asleep is much later. Or advanced sleep phase syndrome patients may complain of an inability to stay asleep or early morning awakening. Shift workers may complain of difficulty falling asleep during the day. A degree of sleep state misperception (paradoxical insomnia) might be suspected based on an incongruous relationship between the perceived amount of sleep obtained and the absence of significant clinical consequences from the lack of sleep.

Sleep habits may perpetuate insomnia. Therefore, it is important to ask what time patients lie down in bed, what time they think they fall asleep, when they awaken in the night, and what time they get out of bed. It is also helpful to know what activities they engage in prior to sleep and while in bed. These activities can exacerbate the sleep difficulties. Sometimes hours are spent lying in bed but not sleeping, and this activity may solidify the negative association of the bed with tossing, turning, and the inability to fall asleep. Spending prolonged amounts of time in bed can be self-defeating for patients, can loosen their association between the bed and sleep, and may result in less sleep consolidation. Asking about clock watching or reading in bed can help identify potential targets to address in insomnia management.

Movement disorders and parasomnias

Patients may describe abnormal behaviors or sensations just prior to sleep. A patient may note restlessness that can delay sleep onset. This restless sensation can result in an insufficient amount of sleep, contributing to sleepiness. One should ask about the classic symptoms of restless legs syndrome that include an uncomfortable sensation or urge to move the legs (and sometimes the arms) which is worse in the evening, occurs when sedentary, improves with movement, and can prevent sleep onset. If these symptoms are present, it is important to identify exacerbating factors, such as neuropathy, renal failure, iron deficiency, and medications/substances. Use of substances that are likely to worsen symptoms, such as stimulants, caffeine, and psychotropic medications, should be explored.

Hypnogogic and hypnopompic hallucinations can suggest the diagnosis of narcolepsy, as mentioned above. Some other events that occur temporally around sleep include sleep paralysis and myoclonic jerks. Sleep paralysis can be a normal event but if it occurs with frequency, it can be pathological. Similarly, myoclonic jerks are normal phenomena but when the patient is overly concerned with them, then they may cause anxiety and reassurance is necessary.

Abnormal behaviors during sleep, or parasomnias, are quite common in childhood and have a familial predisposition. The most important information to obtain is a good description of the event at night, and, at times, home videos may be helpful. One should determine when in the sleep period these activities occur. This can help distinguish the non-rapid eye movement (non-REM) from the rapid eye movement (REM) parasomnias. Events that occur closer to sleep onset and predominate in the first third of the sleep period are more consistent with non-REM parasomnias. Non-REM parasomnias include sleepwalking, sleep eating, night terrors, and confusional arousals. The duration of symptoms and triggers to the behaviors should be determined. Some common triggers include periods of stress and sleep deprivation. Disorders that disrupt sleep, leading to arousals from sleep, can also exacerbate parasomnias. Therefore, the patient should be questioned about events that may disrupt their sleep such as apneas, gasp arousals, or leg movements.

Medication use should also be explored as some medications, notably the non-benzodiazepine hypnotics such as zolpidem, have been associated with sleepwalking. The context of the behaviors can also suggest a diagnosis. For example, confusional arousals are behaviors associated with an arousal and accompanied by some mental confusion. The patient either wakes up more fully from the event or goes back to sleep and has little recall of the event. The presence or absence of recall for the events can also differentiate the diagnosis. In night terrors, patients, usually children, scream or cry out and are often inconsolable. However, there is no recall of the event, even immediately after, whereas in nightmare disorder, the disturbing dreams are usually remembered.

Rapid eye movement parasomnias tend to occur later in the sleep period. Again, disruptors of sleep may precipitate the events, and therefore patients should be questioned regarding other sleep disorders. Nightmares should be explored for dream content and underlying stress or events that may be causing the nightmares. If REM sleep behavior

disorder is suspected, understanding the dream content is helpful. Often, the dream content has been described as defensive, where the individual is fending off attackers or trying to protect himself or a loved one.

A primary differential diagnosis for parasomnias is seizures. A prior history of seizures, history of major head injury, or ongoing febrile illness may increase the chances of seizure being the cause of the nocturnal behavior. Tongue biting and loss of continence are associated with seizures, but not typically with most parasomnias.

Determining the consequences of the parasomnias is necessary. Safety is of paramount importance. If a patient has put themselves or others at risk with their sleep-related activities then it is important to discuss ways to limit the events and to prevent injury by creating a safe environment.

⚡ CAUTION

It is imperative to assess patient safety in the setting of the sleep complaints. Assess whether the individual presents a safety threat to themselves, bed partners, or the public. If so, ensure that the patient and family are adequately counseled and that appropriate precautionary measures are taken.

Past medical history

Knowledge of previous diagnoses of sleep disorders and their management is helpful to the current evaluation. But it is also important to consider the rest of the medical history (Table 2.2). Co-existing medical conditions can contribute to sleep disorders or have a higher prevalence in certain disorders.

Eye, ear, nose, and throat issues can lead to sleep disorders. For example, blind patients may have difficulty following typical circadian rhythms and schedules due to a free-running circadian rhythm sleep disorder. Chronic sinusitis, nasal polyps, and a deviated nasal septum may all be associated with snoring, sleepiness, and sleep apnea.

Cardiovascular diseases, particularly hypertension, are clearly associated with the presence of sleep-disordered breathing. Congestive heart failure has been associated with central sleep apnea syndrome. Cerebrovascular accidents have been associated with both obstructive and central sleep apnea.

Table 2.2 Key features of the medical history in common sleep disorders

Diagnosis	Chief complaint	Key features of the medical history
Obstructive sleep apnea	Excessive sleepiness, loud snoring	Loud snoring, witnessed apneas, gasp or choke arousals, morning headaches, unintentional dozing, unrefreshing naps
Central sleep apnea	Excessive sleepiness, fragmented sleep	Pauses in breathing, disrupted sleep, associated with medications (e.g. narcotics), increased risk at higher altitudes, may be associated with other medical conditions (e.g. central nervous system abnormalities, heart failure)
Narcolepsy	Excessive sleepiness	Cataplexy, sleep paralysis, hypnogogic or hypnopompic hallucinations, sleep attacks, unintentional dozing, refreshing naps, symptom onset in adolescence
Idiopathic hypersomnia	Excessive sleepiness	Associated with normal or prolonged sleep duration, unrefreshing naps
Delayed sleep phase syndrome	Excessive sleepiness and/or insomnia	Difficulty falling asleep at a conventional bedtime, sleeping in late when given the opportunity, "night owl" tendency, less difficulty on vacation, symptom onset in adolescence
Advanced sleep phase syndrome	Excessive sleepiness and/or insomnia	Difficulty staying awake in the evening, difficulty sleeping later in the mornings with early morning awakening, "early bird" tendency, symptom onset in middle age
Shift work sleep disorder	Excessive sleepiness and/or insomnia	Sleepiness during an unconventional work period, difficulty falling asleep during the day, working rotating or night shift
Chronic insufficient sleep syndrome	Excessive sleepiness	Regularly obtaining a decreased amount of sleep, unintentional dozing, refreshing naps, may sleep more on vacation
Recurrent hypersomnia	Excessive sleepiness	Prolonged sleep periods, cyclical nature, associated with menstrual cycle, associated with hyperphagia and hypersexuality
Hypersomnia due to medication, substance, or medical condition	Excessive sleepiness	Symptoms are temporally related to the underlying condition, may result from medication use or substance use/abuse, thyroid disorders, mood disorders
Primary insomnia	Insomnia	Long standing, usually present since childhood, no clear trigger, inability to nap, no hypersomnia *per se*
Psychophysiological insomnia	Insomnia	Pervasive thoughts regarding sleep and sleep difficulties, heightened arousal in bed, often improved on vacation, may be perpetuated by certain behaviors such as clock watching
Paradoxical insomnia	Insomnia	Difficulty falling and/or staying asleep, extreme sleep complaints, amount of sleep reported is incongruent with physiological symptoms
Co-morbid insomnia	Insomnia	Difficulty falling and/or staying asleep, sleep is disrupted, there is another underlying disorder contributing to this insomnia (e.g. anxiety, thyroid disease, medications, substance abuse)

(continued)

Table 2.2 (Continued)

Diagnosis	Chief complaint	Key features of the medical history
Confusional arousal	Abnormal behavior in sleep	Confusion or abnormal or inappropriate behavior upon arousal from sleep, memory of the event may be impaired, more common in children and young adults
Sleepwalking	Sleepwalking	Complex behaviors during sleep, more prominent in earlier part of the night, impaired memory of the event
Night terror	Screaming at night	Screaming at night, little to no recall of the event, difficult to arouse, most common in children
Rapid eye movement sleep behavior disorder	Abnormal behaviors at night	Dream enactment, often violent dreams, usually no aggression or violent behavior during the day, more common in middle-aged and older men, associated with neurodegenerative disorders, may injure self or bed partner
Restless legs syndrome	Restlessness at bedtime or insomnia	Uncomfortable sensation or urge to move the legs (sometimes arms), worse when sedentary, worse in the evening, improved with movement, can prevent sleep onset, can be exacerbated by medications and other medical conditions (e.g. anemia)

Data suggest a relationship between nocturnal asthma and sleep apnea. Also, persistent or poorly controlled respiratory symptoms can disrupt sleep, leading to either insomnia or daytime sleepiness.

Gastrointestinal diseases have been correlated with specific sleep disorders. A relationship between nocturnal gastroesophageal reflux disease and sleep apnea has been reported. Gastrointestinal diseases can also result in vitamin or mineral deficiencies, such as iron deficiency, which can contribute to restless legs syndrome and periodic limb movement disorder.

The endocrine system has multiple influences on sleep and vice versa. Endocrinopathies have been correlated with sleep disorders. For example, untreated thyroid disorders can result in sleepiness or insomnia. Other endocrinopathies, such as the metabolic syndrome, have been associated with sleep-disordered breathing. Hormonal changes can contribute to insomnia symptoms: menopausal women have increased likelihood of insomnia which may be exacerbated by hot flashes. In men, low testosterone levels have been noted in some patients with obstructive sleep apnea syndrome.

Rheumatological problems can contribute to chronic fatigue or sleepiness. Chronic pain disrupts sleep and treatment of chronic pain with opiate medications can contribute to both obstructive and central apnea syndromes and sleepiness. Genitourinary problems commonly cause difficulty

with sleep. In older men, prostate problems may lead to urinary frequency with sleep disruption. However, frequent nocturia may also be a symptom of obstructive sleep apnea. Renal disease can contribute to restless legs syndrome. Furthermore, dialysis regimens have been associated with worsening of obstructive sleep apnea syndrome.

Hematological disorders may contribute to sleep disorders. Iron deficiency anemia is associated with restless legs syndrome (RLS). Treatments for hematological malignancies can cause fatigue and sleepiness.

Neurological disorders have been associated with concurrent sleep disorders. Intracranial abnormalities such as Chiari malformation have been linked to central sleep apnea syndrome. Traumatic brain injury has been associated with hypersomnia. Neurodegenerative disorders can contribute to REM sleep behavior disorder (RBD), and in fact, the diagnosis of RBD can predate the diagnosis of neurodegenerative disorders by 10 or more years. Furthermore, dementia can be associated with insomnia, sleepiness, and circadian rhythm abnormalities.

Psychiatric diseases and sleep disorders are closely linked. Psychiatric disorders, particularly depression, have been associated with untreated sleep apnea. In children, there has been a demonstrable correlation between the presence of snoring and sleep apnea and the diagnosis of attention deficit hyperactivity disorder. Mood disorders, such as anxiety, and insomnia often complicate each other with a bidirectional relationship. Other psychiatric disorders, e.g. schizophrenia, can lead to insomnia and be associated with circadian rhythm sleep disorders, such as irregular sleep-wake disorder.

Medications

A complete list of prescription and non-prescription medications, vitamins, and supplements should be obtained. Knowledge of current and prior sleep aid and supplement use, their dosing schedule, efficacy, and side-effects is particularly helpful in management and directing further therapy. It is important to assess for how long current medications have been taken, what they are being taken for, and the timing of the medications during the day.

Many medications can cause sleepiness as an undesired side-effect. Narcotics, benzodiazepines, certain antidepressants, and antihistamines are some key culprits. However, muscle relaxants and antispasmodic agents can also contribute to sleepiness. Medication use or withdrawal can also lead to sleepiness or disrupted sleep.

Insomnia may be a key side-effect of many medications. Stimulant medications can delay sleep onset undesirably, particularly when taken in the afternoon or evening. Withdrawing from sedative medications can lead to rebound insomnia. Certain antidepressants are stimulating and others sedating; thus, altering timing of medication administration may help with sleep issues. Some nasal decongestants may have stimulant effects, which patients may not realize.

Many substances, including the selective serotonin reuptake inhibitors (SSRIs), can cause "pseudo-RBD" which mimics RBD but improves or resolves with discontinuation of these substances. This group of medications, as well as stimulant medications, may also cause or worsen RLS and periodic limb movements. Medications such as the non-benzodiazepine sedative-hypnotics (e.g. zolpidem) can also contribute to or worsen sleepwalking.

Medication allergies

A complete history includes medication allergies. It is obviously imperative to know these allergies prior to prescribing medications to manage patient's medical problems.

Social history

The use and timing of stimulants, caffeine, sleep aids, and other substances that can affect sleep provide helpful information, as mentioned above. The amount of caffeine used to combat sleepiness can suggest the severity of hypersomnolence, but overuse of caffeine can also lead to insomnia or other issues with sleep, including RLS or periodic limb movement disorder. Caffeine use may perpetuate poor sleep habits, chronic insufficient sleep, and circadian rhythm disorders. Therefore, it is particularly important to determine the amount and timing of caffeine ingestion over the day.

Both legal and illegal substances can affect sleep, by either increasing or decreasing the propensity to sleep, whether desired or not. Some patients have used substances to self-manage their sleep issues. For example, nicotine may be used to combat sleepiness during the day, and nicotine withdrawal during the night may contribute to fragmented sleep. Patients may depend on alcohol to manage insomnia issues. Alcohol may help induce sleep but then leads to more sleep disruption as the night progresses. Alcohol can also worsen underlying sleep apnea and contribute to pseudo-RBD.

The presence of a bed partner, children, or pets that may influence sleep quality should be determined. Considering bed partners and household members is also important when assessing safety in patients with parasomnias. Furthermore, knowing a patient's work or school schedule and the effect on their sleep schedule can help with the evaluation, particularly as shift work has become more common in our society. Active stressors are likely to influence sleep. In patients suffering from insomnia, it is particularly important to identify social stressors that are contributing to the sleeping problem and to try to help the patient alleviate those factors.

Family history

The family history helps elicit a genetic or environmental factor to sleep complaints. Because many sleep disorders have a familial component, inquiring about the presence of sleep problems in family members is helpful. For example, narcolepsy tends to be familial, as does sleepwalking. Sleep-disordered breathing has a propensity to run in families, which may be due in part to the genetics of weight and facial structure. Family members with similar diagnoses who respond well to treatment, such as those who use positive pressure for obstructive sleep apnea, may provide support for the newly diagnosed patient.

There also may be a familial propensity to insomnia, perhaps related to the genetics of mood disorders. In addition, fatal familial insomnia is a very rare inheritable prion disease causing insomnia and a range of other neurological symptoms.

Restless legs syndrome tends to be present in other family members. Also, sleepwalking may occur in other first-degree relatives. A family history of dream enactment should prompt questions regarding Parkinson's disease and neurodegenerative disorders because RBD symptoms often predate the diagnosis of those neurological disorders.

Review of systems

Each organ system should be reviewed. As mentioned in the past medical history section, sleep disorders can lead to systemic manifestations. Untreated sleep disorders can manifest with a multitude of symptoms involving almost any organ system. Likewise, various co-existing medical problems can contribute to sleep problems. Sleep disorders can exacerbate or be exacerbated by such issues as weight gain, thyroid disorders, cardiovascular diseases, cognitive decline, and mood disorders. Nocturnal reflux symptoms could suggest a diagnosis of sleep apnea. Symptoms of rigidity or mental decline can support the exploration for neurodegenerative problems and the possibility of REM behavior sleep disorder. The presence of hot flashes can suggest hormonal changes as the trigger for insomnia.

Supplemental information

Beyond direct history taking, questionnaires can be helpful; these will be covered in detail later in this book. They can help assess factors such as sleep quality and daytime sleepiness. The Epworth Sleepiness Scale can help quantify a person's degree of sleepiness by asking about sleep propensity in everyday situations. The STOP-BANG questionnaire was developed to simplify the evaluation of obstructive sleep apnea through a brief series of questions and physical exam findings. Sleep logs and sleep diaries may also provide valuable data regarding sleep schedules and trends. While this supplemental information can be helpful, it is important

not to rely solely on questionnaires and logs because patients may not fill them out correctly or their use may not be pertinent to certain populations.

The physical examination

Once a thorough history is obtained, a comprehensive physical examination helps to establish potential etiologies for the sleep complaints. Key portions of the physical examination can help confirm the diagnosis (Table 2.3).

General factors such as appearance, age, gender, and race can all suggest more specific diagnoses. A disheveled appearance may suggest an underlying psychiatric disorder or severe fatigue from chronic insomnia. As mentioned previously, the prevalence and presentation of sleep disorders have

Table 2.3 Important physical examination elements in the sleep patient

Examination element	What to examine
Vital signs	Heart rate, blood pressure, height, weight, respiratory rate, pulse oximetry
General appearance	Gender, race, age, body weight
Head and neck	Inspection, palpation for lymphadenopathy, palpation of thyroid gland
Nasoooropharynx	Nasal mucosal edema, nasal polyps, Mallampati classification, dental occlusion, tongue size
Cardiovascular system	Heart sounds, rhythm and rate, edema
Respiratory system	Breath sounds, respiratory effort, chest excursion
Gastrointestinal system	Abdominal masses or protuberant abdomen
Musculoskeletal	Joint abnormalities or swelling, tenderness
Skin	Rashes, color, trauma, bruising, signs of abuse
Neurological system	Deficits, localization, strength, gait, speech, thought
Psychiatric	Affect, behavior, thought content

gender and age differences. Racial differences are notable as well; for example, narcolepsy has a greater prevalence in the Japanese population.

Vital signs are important in assessing patient stability and risk factors associated with sleep disorders. Hypertension may be documented in a patient with sleep-disordered breathing because of the potential influence of untreated sleep apnea on blood pressure. Abnormal pulse oximetry suggests hypoventilation, underlying lung conditions, or cardiovascular issues. Height and weight measurements are used to determine Body Mass Index (BMI) with obesity defined by a BMI greater than 30. Central obesity, in particular, with an elevated waist-to-hip ratio, identifies patients at significant risk for sleep apnea.

The head should be inspected for trauma and for abnormalities. Craniofacial abnormalities or syndromes, such as Down's syndrome, have been associated with obstructive sleep apnea (OSA). Determining jaw position by viewing the patient from the side can support the suspicion of sleep-disordered breathing, with retrognathia or micrognathia being risk factors for OSA. Evidence of prior head trauma suggests a possible etiology for sleep complaints.

The upper airway is evaluated for potential sites of upper airway narrowing. The nasal examination may reveal obstructions which can contribute to snoring and sleep-disordered breathing. These abnormalities include a deviated nasal septum, nasal congestion, and nasal polyps. A large tongue, also known as macroglossia, or visible scalloping along the tongue support the presence of sleep apnea. The oropharynx is inspected for airway crowdedness (e.g. Mallampati class 3–4 airway) which has been associated with an increased risk of sleep apnea.

The Mallampati classification was initially developed to stratify risk for difficult airway intubations with higher classifications indicating more difficulty. However, with the modified Mallampati classification (Figure 2.1), class 3 and 4 airways have also been associated with an increased prevalence of obstructive sleep apnea. Obvious obstructions such as significantly enlarged tonsils support an anatomical abnormality contributing to sleep apnea. Dentition should be evaluated. Molar classification helps with assessment of sleep apnea (see Table 2.4). Severe overjet, or class II

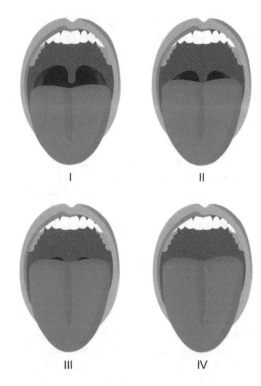

I   II

III   IV

Figure 2.1 The modified Mallampati classification. From: http://en.wikipedia.org/wiki/Mallampati_ score. This file is licensed under the Creative Commons Attribution-Share Alike 3.0 Unported license. Permission is granted to copy, distribute and/or modify this document under the terms of the GNU Free Documentation License, Version 1.2 or any later version published by the Free Software Foundation.

Table 2.4 Molar occlusion classification

Class	Findings
Normal	Normal alignment of the upper and lower first molars and normal alignment of teeth
Class I	Normal relationship between the upper and lower teeth and jaw but with the presence of crowding, teeth misalignment, or cross-bite
Class II	The lower first molar is more behind the top first molar than normal. The chin may be recessed
Class III	The lower first molar is more forward of the top first molar than normal. Chin may protrude outward

malocclusion, has been correlated with severity of sleep apnea. Also, poor or absent dentition would preclude the use of an oral mandibular advancement device for treatment of sleep apnea. Changes consistent with bruxism such as flattening and wearing down of dental surfaces should be noted.

Neck circumference measurements of greater than 16 inches in women and 17 inches in men have been associated with an increased propensity for sleep apnea. The neck should be palpated for lymphadenopathy and thyroid abnormalities which could suggest etiologies for sleep complaints (i.e. lymphoma causing night sweats or fatigue). Lesions of the neck, such as goiter, can cause extrinsic airway compression, resulting in sleep-disordered breathing.

The cardiovascular exam includes auscultation for arrhythmias, murmurs, and abnormal heart sounds. Arrhythmias may be associated with sleep apnea. Additional or pronounced heart sounds may be heard in patients with pulmonary hypertension or congestive heart failure, which also may be linked to sleep-disordered breathing.

The respiratory evaluation includes listening for abnormal breath sounds such as wheezes or crackles, which may suggest an underlying obstructive or restrictive process, respectively. Respiratory weakness may also be assessed based on minimal diaphragmatic excursion or asymmetrical chest expansion.

The gastrointestinal exam should include palpation and inspection. Factors such as abdominal obesity or severe ascites support suspicion for sleep apnea.

The musculoskeletal evaluation includes inspecting for abnormalities that would suggest a rheumatological disorder or determining areas of pain that may contribute to sleep disruption. Assessment for trigger points can support the diagnosis of fibromyalgia, which may exacerbate or be exacerbated by underlying sleep disorders. Lower extremity edema, cyanosis, or digital clubbing suggest hypoxia or underlying lung or cardiac disease, including inadequately controlled congestive heart failure.

The skin should be inspected for signs of bruising or injury from abnormal nocturnal behaviors. Intravenous drug use can be suspected based on skin markings. Pallor could suggest anemia or lack of sufficient light exposure.

The neurological examination includes an assessment of motor strength and reflexes. Localizing lesions can suggest prior stroke or other neurological abnormalities, which have a higher incidence of sleep apnea. Abnormalities in gait and speech could suggest intracranial lesions. Sequelae of poor or insufficient sleep, such as insomnia and sleep apnea, can include memory and concentration issues. Signs of neurodegenerative disorders and dementia should be examined since they have been associated with REM sleep behavior disorder and circadian rhythm abnormalities.

The psychiatric evaluation includes an assessment of the patient's mood and affect, such as anxiety or blunted affect. These mood issues may be the result of or the cause of sleep complaints. Appropriateness of behavior, speech, responses to questions, and thought content can support diagnosis of co-existing psychiatric disorders.

★ TIPS AND TRICKS

Because of the many questions needed to take a good sleep history, it is often helpful to create a template of important questions and issues to address during the evaluation.

Conclusion

In conclusion, sleep disorders are common. Sleep complaints represent a broad group of disorders resulting from myriad factors; therefore, a comprehensive history and physical examination are necessary for an adequate assessment of potential sleep disorders. It is important to consider the patient in the context of age and gender because specific sleep disorders are more common in certain patient populations. Co-existing medical problems can lead to or result from certain sleep disorders. Many medications affect sleep and may cause either daytime sleepiness or nocturnal insomnia. Social factors such as work schedules, caffeine,nicotine, and alcohol use, and stressors have sleep-related implications. Sleep disorders often have a genetic or familial tendency. Considering key aspects of the sleep history, with focused questions based on the primary sleep complaint, helps guide the evaluation of sleep issues. Appropriate diagnosis of sleep disorders and complicating factors leads to successful management of patients, with overall benefits to their health and well-being.

Further reading

Allen RP, Walters AS, Montplaisir J, et al. Restless legs syndrome prevalence and impact: REST general population study. *Arch Intern Med* 2005; **165**(11): 1286–92.

American Academy of Sleep Medicine. *International Classification of Sleep Disorders*, 2nd edn. Westchester, IL: American Academy of Sleep Medicine, 2005.

Chervin RD, Ruzicka DL, Giordani BJ, et al. Sleep-disordered breathing, behavior, and cognition in children before and after adenotonsillectomy. *Pediatrics* 2006; **177**(4); e769–78.

Davies RJ, Ali NJ, Stradling JR. Neck circumference and other clinical features in the diagnosis of the obstructive sleep apnoea syndrome. *Thorax* 1992; **47**(2): 101–5.

Hiremath AS, Hillman DR, James AL, Noffsinger WJ, Platt PR, Singer SL. Relationship between difficult tracheal intubation and obstructive sleep apnoea. *Br J Anaesth* 1998; **80**(5): 606–11.

Johns MW. A new method for measuring daytime sleepiness: the Epworth sleepiness scale. *Sleep* 1991; **14**(6): 540–5.

Miyao E, Noda A, Miyao M, Yasuma F, Inafuku S. The role of malocclusion in non-obese patients with obstructive sleep apnea syndrome. *Intern Med* 2008; **47**(18): 1573–8.

Peppard PE, Young T, Palta M, Skatrud J. Prospective study of the association between sleep-disordered breathing and hypertension. *N Engl J Med* 2000; **342**(19): 1378–84.

Poceta JS. Zolpidem ingestion, automatisms, and sleep driving: a clinical and legal case series. *J Clin Sleep Med* 2011; **7**(6): 632–8.

Schenck CH, Bundlie SR, Mahowald MW. Delayed emergence of a parkinsonian disorder in 38% of 29 older men initially diagnosed with idiopathic rapid eye movement sleep behaviour disorder. *Neurology* 1996; **46**: 388–93.

Silva GE, Vana KD, Goodwin JL, Sherrill DL, Quan SF. Identification of patients with sleep disordered breathing: comparing the four-variable screening tool, STOP, STOP-Bang, and Epworth Sleepiness Scales. *J Clin Sleep Med* 2011; **7**(5): 467–72.

Somers VK, White DP, Amin R, et al. Sleep apnea and cardiovascular disease: an American Heart Association/American College of Cardiology Foundation Scientific Statement from the American Heart Association Council for High Blood Pressure Research Professional Education Committee, Council on Clinical Cardiology, Stroke Council, and Council on Cardiovascular Nursing. *J Am Coll Cardiol* 2008; **52**(8): 686–717.

Tsai SC. Excessive sleepiness. *Clin Chest Med* 2010; **31**(2): 341–51.

3

Subjective and Objective Sleep Testing

Martha E. Billings, MD[1] and Nathaniel F. Watson, MD, MS[2]

[1]Department of Medicine, Division of Pulmonary Critical Care, University of Washington, UW Medicine Sleep Center, Harborview Medical Center, USA
[2]Department of Neurology, University of Washington, UW Medicine Sleep Center, Harborview Medical Center, USA

Introduction

Sleep disorders are common co-morbidities in patients with neurological disorders. Obstructive sleep apnea (OSA) is a major modifiable risk factor for stroke, seen in up to 80% of stroke patients. Insomnia is observed in patients who suffer from Parkinson's disease, multiple sclerosis, chronic headache, and dementia, frequently exacerbating the clinical picture. Restless legs syndrome (RLS) has been noted in peripheral neuropathy, radiculopathy, Parkinson's disease, multiple sclerosis, Charcot–Marie–Tooth disease, and spinal cord lesions. Rapid eye movement (REM) sleep behavior disorder (RBD) is associated with synucleinopathies such as multisystem atrophy, Parkinson's disease and Lewy body dementia. Traumatic brain injury can result in sleepiness, insomnia, and circadian rhythm dysfunction.

Assessing for sleep disorders includes subjective tests exploring the patient's perceived sleepiness, difficulty sleeping, sleep quality and symptom severity as well as objective diagnostic testing. Many sleep disorders can be diagnosed by patient interview and physical examination alone, but subjective and objective testing may be useful to further quantify the disorder and assess treatment responsiveness.

In this chapter we will describe a few of the more commonly used subjective assessments to evaluate sleepiness, OSA risk, insomnia presence and severity, and RLS as well as measures used to evaluate quality of life in sleep disorders and sleep quality, summarized in Table 3.1. Most of these questionnaires are simple to administer and interpret and can be used in the office. We will also discuss the most common objective sleep tests including polysomnography (PSG), the Multiple Sleep Latency Test (MSLT), the Maintenance of Wakefulness Test (MWT), actigraphy, and the Suggested Immobilization Test (SIT), summarized in Table 3.2. These tests are typically performed in a sleep laboratory and interpreted by a sleep specialist. The costs, complexity, and inconvenience to the patient vary with each test so selecting the correct test is crucial.

Subjective testing

A simple, structured, and useful tool to evaluate your patient's sleep is the sleep diary. Over the course of 2 weeks, patients report bedtime, wake time, rise time, naps, sleep latency, and nighttime awakenings (see Appendix 1). This enables the practitioner to get a sense of the patient's circadian rhythm and weekday and weekend sleep habits. These diaries are very useful for insomnia, hypersomnia, shift work sleep disorder, circadian rhythm disorders, and insufficient sleep syndrome. Also useful is the Sleep Habits Questionnaire (SHQ).[1] This tool establishes typical sleep patterns, circadian rhythms, and sleep difficulties. Unlike the sleep diary, the questionnaire can be completed during the first office visit. The SHQ has been used in multiple studies as well as clinically to characterize sleep.

Sleep Medicine in Neurology, First Edition. Edited by Douglas B. Kirsch.
© 2014 John Wiley & Sons, Ltd. Published 2014 by John Wiley & Sons, Ltd.

Table 3.1 Subjective sleep tests

Measurement	Subjective test	References	Appendices
Circadian rhythm	SHQ, sleep diary	1	1 (diary)
Sleepiness	ESS, KSS, SSS	2, 5 and 6	2 (SSS)
OSA screening	Berlin Questionnaire, STOP-BANG, four-variable screening tool	11, 13, 15	
Patient-reported outcome	FOSQ, SAQLI, PSQI	9, 16, 17	
Insomnia	ISI, sleep diary	18	3 (ISI)
RLS	International RLS rating scale	20	

Table 3.2 Objective sleep tests components

	EEG	EOG	EMG	Respiratory/cardiac	Used for diagnosis
PSG	X	X	X	X	All SDB/seizures/parasomnias/RBD
OCST				X	OSA only
MSLT	X	X	X (chin)	+/– (EKG)	Narcolepsy
MWT	X	X	X (chin)	+/– (EKG)	Sleepiness
SIT	+/–		X		RLS

X, included; +/–, optional.

Sleepiness

The most commonly used measure of subjective sleepiness is the Epworth Sleepiness Scale (ESS) developed in 1991.[2] The ESS includes eight items describing propensity to fall asleep in certain situations on a scale of zero (would never doze) to three (high chance of dozing). Out of 24, a score greater than 10 is considered abnormal. The ESS is routinely used in sleep clinics to assess for the severity of daytime sleepiness and measure the treatment effects of continuous positive airway pressure (CPAP) for OSA, now a standard adopted by Medicare. Very high scores on the ESS (>15) are associated with narcolepsy, idiopathic hypersomnia, and severe OSA. ESS scores do not correlate well with the MSLT,[3] an objective measure of sleep propensity, or with the Apnea-Hypopnea Index (AHI) from PSG.[4]

Two other simpler measures of sleep propensity are the Stanford Sleepiness Scale (SSS) developed in

1972[5] and the Karolinska Sleepiness Scale (KSS) formulated in 1990.[6] Both questionnaires ask subjects to rate their current level of sleepiness and likelihood of falling asleep. Both can be used repeatedly over the day. The SSS asks subjects to pick one of seven statements rating sleepiness from one, "feeling active and vital; alert; wide awake" to seven, "lost struggle to remain awake" (see Appendix 2). The KSS has a scale from one (very alert) to nine (very sleepy) similar to a visual analogue scale. These scales are well validated and correlate with objective sleep measures such as alpha activity on electroencephalogram (EEG) and performance.[7,8] They are commonly used in research settings evaluating shift work sleep disorder, as well as in the transportation industry. Because the KSS and SSS are affected by circadian factors, they are less useful for assessing treatment responsiveness and chronic sleepiness.

The Functional Outcomes of Sleep Questionnaire (FOSQ), a 30-item self-administered questionnaire, evaluates the impact of excessive sleepiness on activities of daily life.[9] The FOSQ is validated in populations with OSA and can identify those with sleep disorders. It includes five factor analysis-derived subscales: activity level, vigilance, intimacy, general

---

⚠ CAUTION

The ESS does not correlate with objective sleepiness measures and is not a good screening tool for identification of OSA.

productivity, and social outcome. Subjects are asked if sleepiness interferes with performing a given task; responses range from one (extreme difficulty) to four (no difficulty), with greater scores indicating less impact of sleepiness on daily life. A score greater than 18 is considered normal. A shorter 10-item version can be used in instances requiring brevity.[10] The FOSQ is a useful clinical measure of patient-reported outcome.

Obstructive sleep apnea screening tests

Given the high prevalence of OSA, a simple screening tool to identify high-risk individuals for further evaluation is helpful. The Berlin Questionnaire (BQ) is one of the most widely adopted OSA screening tools. It has 10 items comprising three sections: presence of snoring and witnessed apneas, consequences of OSA including daytime sleepiness, and physical characteristics such as hypertension and Body Mass Index (BMI). Scoring positive in two or more categories is considered high risk for OSA. This well-validated OSA screening instrument has a robust positive predictive value of 0.89 and is often used in primary care and preoperative settings.[11] However, its specificity and sensitivity lag behind newer screening tools.[12]

More recently, simpler screening tools have been developed. The STOP questionnaire has been validated in surgical patients and consists of just four yes/no questions. STOP is a mnemonic for Snoring, Tired, Observed stopping breathing, and elevated blood Pressure. The STOP questionnaire has been incorporated with the BANG clinical evaluation for OSA risk, a mnemonic for BMI >35 kg/m2, Age >50 years, Neck circumference >40 cm, and male Gender. Answering "yes" to three or more of the eight items in the STOP-BANG model reflects an increased risk for OSA.[13] The higher the STOP-BANG total, the higher the probability of more severe OSA.[14] The four-variable screening instrument gives points for BMI category, blood pressure category, four points for snoring and male gender.[15] A cut-off of 14 is positive for OSA risk. Using data from the Sleep Heart Health Study, the four-variable screening tool had the highest specificity for severe OSA, while the STOP-BANG had higher sensitivity.[12] Because this is a screening, and not diagnostic, tool, sensitivity has a greater value than specificity, suggesting the longer STOP-BANG is the preferred iteration of this instrument.

The Calgary Sleep Apnea Quality of Life Index (SAQLI) is an interviewer-administered questionnaire evaluating the consequences of sleep apnea on daily activities, emotional functioning, social interactions, and symptoms over the past 4 weeks.[16] If subjects are receiving treatment for OSA, an additional subscale includes treatment-related symptoms. Subjects' responses range from one ("all of the time/large problem/large amount") to seven ("none of the time/not a problem/none") for 56 items. A greater SAQLI score indicates less of an impact of the effects of OSA on quality of life.

Sleep quality

Evaluating the perceived quality of sleep is important for assessing sleep disorders, chronic disease, and mental illness. Poor sleep quality is associated with worse perceived general health, work absenteeism, and increased healthcare utilization. The Pittsburg Sleep Quality Index (PSQI) is a 19-item self-administered questionnaire assessing sleep quality over the past month.[17] It was developed for use in psychiatry but has been widely adopted in sleep medicine. Scores range from 0 to 21, with higher scores reflecting worse sleep. A cut-off score of above five has a specificity and sensitivity for sleep disorders of over 85%. The PSQI does not correlate well with the ESS or objective sleep measurements such as PSG or actigraphy, but does associate with psychological symptoms.[4]

Insomnia

Insomnia is highly prevalent, affecting up to 33% of adults. The Insomnia Severity Index (ISI) has been used to quantify the frequency, severity, and impact of insomnia and evaluate treatment responsiveness. It is a seven-item scale including daytime and nighttime symptoms; scores range from 0 to 28 – less than 7 indicates no insomnia, more than 21 severe insomnia (see Appendix 3). It has established validity and reliability;

a cut-off score of 10 in a community sample had good specificity and sensitivity for insomnia.[18]

Restless legs syndrome

Restless legs syndrome (RLS) is a common disorder with a prevalence of 4% in the general population. Assessing for RLS can be done with a single screening question: "When you try to relax in the evening or sleep at night, do you ever have unpleasant, restless feelings in your legs that can be relieved by walking or movement?" This question has sensitivity and specificity for RLS.[19] The International RLS Rating Scale is a 10-item scale that characterizes RLS symptoms, frequency, and severity.[20] Responses range from zero (never) to four (very severe); a score of less than 10 reflects mild RLS, greater than 31 is categorized as severe RLS.[21]

Objective sleep testing

Polysomnography

The polysomnogram (PSG) is the gold standard test to objectively evaluate sleep disorders and physiology. An in-laboratory PSG includes limited EEG (central and occipital leads using standard 10–20 locations) to determine sleep stage and assess for arousals. More detailed EEG montages can be obtained to evaluate

for sleep-related seizure and complex parasomnias. The electrooculogram (EOG) measures eye movements and is used to determine REM sleep. Chin, leg, and sometimes arm electromyography (EMG) evaluates muscle tone and limb movements. Respiratory monitoring measuring airflow includes both nasal pressure transducers and thermistors to sense hypopneas and apneas. A microphone detects snoring. Chest and abdominal volume changes are measured via respiratory inductance plethysmography, useful in determining if events are central or obstructive. Electrocardiography (EKG) and pulse oximetry are also standard (see Table 3.2). End-tidal CO_2 or transcutaneous CO_2 is used as needed to evaluate for hypoventilation. Sleep technicians also record observed movements, vocalizations, and body position. The PSG should be performed at an accredited sleep center to ensure standardization and quality control.

The PSG must be scored by a sleep technologist and interpreted by a board-certified sleep physician. The PSG provides detailed information on sleep latency, REM latency, sleep architecture, arousals, awakenings after sleep onset, total sleep time, and sleep efficiency. Video recordings allow assessment of parasomnias. Scoring also includes obstructive and central apneas and hypopneas, limb movements, oximetry, and telemetry data (Figure 3.1).

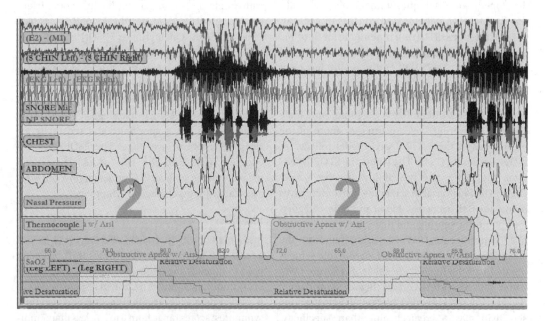

Figure 3.1 Polysomnogram sample. Stage N2 sleep on EEG, chin EMG increased activity with arousal/snore. Nasal pressure and thermocouple demonstrate lack of airflow (apnea); chest and abdominal transducers show obstruction. Oximetry shows relative desaturation with apneic events.

Table 3.3 AASM categories for devices evaluating sleep. A level 1 device requires attendance by a sleep technologist and represents an in-laboratory full PSG

Devices	Channels	EEG/EMG/ EOG	Respiratory	Oximetry	Cardiac
Level 1 (in-lab PSG)	9+	X	Airflow and movement	X	X
Level 2 (unattended)	7+	X	Airflow and movement	X	X
Level 3	4+		Airflow and movement	X	Heart rate or EKG
Level 4	2+		+/– airflow	X	

X, included; +/–, optional.

The rich data of the PSG can allow for evaluation of positional or REM-associated OSA, REM sleep behavior disorder and sleep-related seizures. In-laboratory PSG is indicated for the evaluation of sleep-related breathing disorders, continuous positive airway pressure (CPAP) titration studies, suspected narcolepsy, periodic limb movement disorder, complex, atypical, and injurious parasomnias. It may be indicated in sleep-related seizures not responsive to therapy and in neuromuscular weakness with sleep-related symptoms.[22]

Out-of-center sleep testing (OCST)

The extensive nature of in-laboratory PSG makes home sleep testing appealing for many patients. Nearly all OCST is performed with level 3 devices (Table 3.3), which include only respiratory channels (airflow and effort), oximetry, EKG, and position on some. No EEG, EOG or EMG data are collected as in PSG, thus sleep stage and arousals cannot be determined.

Candidates for OCST for an OSA diagnostic study should have a high pretest probability of OSA based on subjective screening tests, no significant co-morbid medical conditions, and no other suspected sleep disorders. Algorithms for determining which patients should receive in-lab versus home studies vary by sleep center and may not concur with AASM guidelines.[23] Not all level 3 devices are equivalent – the oximetry and airflow sensors differ from device to device and likely yield different sensitivity for diagnosing sleep apnea. A newer classification scheme for devices, updating to levels 1–4, has been developed using the acronym SCOPER (sleep, cardiovascular, oximetry, position, and respiratory), describing the sensors used. Further studies are needed to determine which sensor types (e.g. thermistor, peripheral

arterial tonometry, piezoelectric respiratory effort belts) are minimally required to diagnose OSA with confidence.[24]

With the proper algorithm to identify the ideal patient population and correct device selection, OCST may increase access to sleep testing and be cost-effective. Routine use of type 4 devices (oximetry only) to diagnose OSA is not recommended.[22]

Multiple Sleep Latency Test

Objective quantification of excessive daytime sleepiness is an important step in evaluating complaints of chronic sleepiness. The MSLT measures physiological sleepiness by assessing sleep latency and sleep-onset rapid eye movements (SOREM). This test is indicated to evaluate hypersomnia of central origin and narcolepsy. Starting 90 min to 3 hours after awakening, four to five 20-min napping opportunities are assessed at 2-hours intervals. MSLT protocols are highly standardized.[25] Proper MSLT interpretation requires that the patient not be sleep deprived or taking medications affecting sleep or REM latency (e.g. antihistamines, antidepressants, stimulants). Caffeine should be avoided before and during the test. A urine toxin screen is typically performed to eliminate illicit drug use as a factor influencing the test results. A 2-week sleep diary documenting adequate sleep, a PSG to prove an adequate amount of sleep the night before while assessing for other potential sleep disorders, and treatment of OSA, when present, are important.

Scoring a MSLT focuses on sleep staging while interpretation focuses on mean sleep and REM latency. A mean sleep latency of less than 8 min is abnormal and less than 5 min indicates pathological sleepiness. A MSLT with findings of daytime sleepiness and two or more naps including REM sleep within 15 min of sleep onset is diagnostic for narcolepsy in the correct clinical context.[26]

Maintenance of Wakefulness Test

The MWT, in contrast to the MSLT, evaluates the subject's ability to stay awake in a quiet situation. This test is used to demonstrate response to therapy for excessive daytime sleepiness, especially in professions requiring wakefulness for safety (i.e. pilots, bus drivers, nuclear submarine operators, etc.). The MWT should be performed after effective treatment of underlying sleep disorders and an adequate amount of sleep. Circadian factors, when present, should be accounted for. Typically, the MWT consists of four 40-min periods of sitting in a dark, quiet room. Requiring extreme behavior to stay awake will invalidate the test. For individuals requiring the highest level of safety, staying awake for all four trials is an appropriate expectation.[25] Less than 8 min average sleep latency is considered abnormal. Thus interpretation of the MWT as "normal" can be challenging given the gray zone of sleep latency between 8 and 40 min. Treatment response should show an improvement (increase) in sleep latency.

The utility of the MWT is limited as it may not correlate with real-world job conditions with superimposed circadian disruptions, sleep loss, and environmental factors. Nonetheless, the Federal Aviation Administration requires the MWT for pilots with OSA.[26]

☚ CAUTION

A normal laboratory MWT does not ensure alertness or performance in real-world situations where circadian misalignment and sleep deprivation are commonplace.

Actigraphy

Actigraphy measures activity over time via an accelerometer and has been used to distinguish wake from sleep (Figure 3.2). It provides a real-life assessment of sleep/wake outside the laboratory. Actigraphs are typically worn on the non-dominant wrist like a watch and are most useful to objectively assess circadian rhythm sleep disorders, insomnia, and hypersomnia.[27] Actigraphy is helpful in the objective assessment of adequate sleep in the days leading up to MSLT. Quiet resting with minimal movement may be misinterpreted as sleep and thus actigraphy should be used in combination with a sleep diary. Actigraphy has not been found to correlate well with self-reported sleep habits in standardized questionnaires.[28]

☆ TIPS AND TRICKS

Actigraphy in combination with a sleep diary can help evaluate reports of hypersomnia and insomnia and ensure adequate sleep and circadian alignment in those with excessive daytime sleepiness without evidence of sleep disorders on PSG or MSLT.

Suggested Immobilization Test

The SIT has been used to support the clinical diagnosis of RLS and to provide additional data in uncertain cases. Periodic limb movements during nocturnal wakefulness on PSG are typical of RLS. The SIT provides an alternative, simpler objective test of RLS than PSG, which is not indicated for the diagnosis of RLS. Subjects sit upright in bed in the late evening with their legs outstretched and limit movement in their legs. EMG recording of the anterior tibialis muscle is performed for 1 hour.[29] Subjects may be asked to raise their arm when they feel sensory symptoms or report their discomfort level on a visual analogue scale. A SIT movement index of 40 has an 81% sensitivity and specificity for RLS.[30] A SIT periodic limb movement (PLM) index of 12 is considered diagnostic of RLS but there may be substantial night-to-night variability in symptoms and this cut-off may not be useful in unclear cases.[31] The SIT is not indicated for patients with unequivocal RLS diagnosed clinically.

Conclusion

Sleep disorders are extremely common in the neurology clinic population. Identifying the most specific, sensitive, and cost-effective methods for diagnosing and assessing disease severity and evaluating treatment response is crucial. The subjective and objective tests described should be selected as appropriate for each patient to ensure correct and complete therapy for their sleep disorder. Subjective testing may allow for routine, rapid screening of high-risk populations and repeat evaluation of

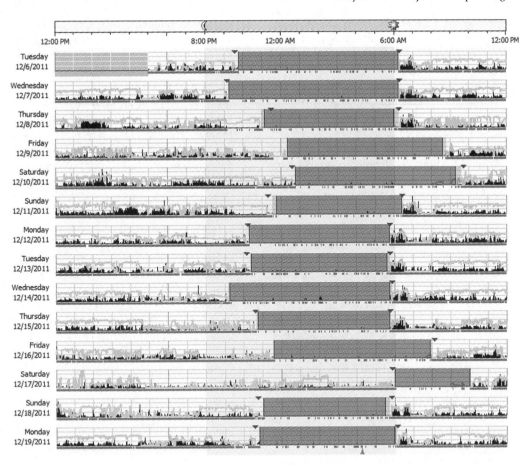

	12:00 PM	8:00 PM	12:00 AM	6:00 AM	12:00 PM

Figure 3.2 Actigraphy sample. Dark blue sections denote time scored as rest (or sleep), black lines indicate wakeful activity, the undulating light grey represents light exposure, small triangles are event markers indicating bedtime and wake time for the individual.

patient-reported outcomes. Objective testing is more resource and time intensive, but is often necessary for precise diagnosis and treatment.

References

1. Sleep Habits Questionnaire. www.jhucct.com/shhs/details/manual/forms/sh/shhshq2.pdf.
2. Johns MW. A new method for measuring daytime sleepiness: the Epworth Sleepiness Scale. *Sleep* 1991; **14**: 540–5.
3. Benbadis SR, Mascha E, Perry MC, Wolgamuth BR, Smolley LA, Dinner DS. Association between the Epworth sleepiness scale and the multiple sleep latency test in a clinical population. *Ann Intern Med* 1999; **130**: 289–92.
4. Buysse DJ, Hall ML, Strollo PJ, et al. Relationships between the Pittsburgh Sleep Quality Index (PSQI), Epworth Sleepiness Scale (ESS), and clinical/polysomnographic measures in a community sample. *J Clin Sleep Med* 2008; **4**: 563–71.
5. Hoddes EDW. The development and use of the Stanford Sleepiness Scale (SSS). *Psychophysiology* 1972; **9**: 150.
6. Akerstedt T, Gillberg M. Subjective and objective sleepiness in the active individual. *Int J Neurosci* 1990; **52**: 29–37.
7. Kaida K, Takahashi M, Akerstedt T, et al. Validation of the Karolinska sleepiness scale against performance and EEG variables. *Clin Neurophysiol* 2006; **117**: 1574–81.
8. Short M, Lack L, Wright H. Does subjective sleepiness predict objective sleep propensity? *Sleep* 2010; **33**: 123–9.

9. Weaver TE, Laizner AM, Evans LK, et al. An instrument to measure functional status outcomes for disorders of excessive sleepiness. *Sleep* 1997; **20**: 835–43.

10. Chasens ER, Ratcliffe SJ, Weaver TE. Development of the FOSQ-10: a short version of the Functional Outcomes of Sleep Questionnaire. *Sleep* 2009; **32**: 915–19.

11. Netzer NC, Stoohs RA, Netzer CM, Clark K, Strohl KP. Using the Berlin Questionnaire to identify patients at risk for the sleep apnea syndrome. *Ann Intern Med* 1999; **131**: 485–91.

12. Silva GE, Vana KD, Goodwin JL, Sherrill DL, Quan SF. Identification of patients with sleep disordered breathing: comparing the four-variable screening tool, STOP, STOP-Bang, and Epworth Sleepiness Scales. *J Clin Sleep Med* 2011; **7**: 467–72.

13. Chung F, Yegneswaran B, Liao P, et al. STOP questionnaire: a tool to screen patients for obstructive sleep apnea. *Anesthesiology* 2008; **108**: 812–21.

14. Farney RJ, Walker BS, Farney RM, Snow GL, Walker JM. The STOP–Bang equivalent model and prediction of severity of obstructive sleep apnea: relation to polysomnographic measurements of the apnea/hypopnea index. *J Clin Sleep Med* 2011; **7**: 459–65B.

15. Takegami M, Hayashino Y, Chin K, et al. Simple four-variable screening tool for identification of patients with sleep-disordered breathing. *Sleep* 2009; **32**: 939–48.

16. Flemons WW, Reimer MA. Development of a disease-specific health-related quality of life questionnaire for sleep apnea. *Am J Respir Crit Care Med* 1998; **158**: 494–503.

17. Buysse DJ, Reynolds CF 3rd, Monk TH, Berman SR, Kupfer DJ. The Pittsburgh Sleep Quality Index: a new instrument for psychiatric practice and research. *Psychiatry Res* 1989; **28**: 193–213.

18. Morin CM, Belleville G, Belanger L, Ivers H. The Insomnia Severity Index: psychometric indicators to detect insomnia cases and evaluate treatment response. *Sleep* 2011; **34**: 601–8.

19. Ferri R, Lanuzza B, Cosentino FI, et al. A single question for the rapid screening of restless legs syndrome in the neurological clinical practice. *Eur J Neurol* 2007; **14**: 1016–21.

20. Walters AS, LeBrocq C, Dhar A, et al. Validation of the International Restless Legs Syndrome Study Group rating scale for restless legs syndrome. *Sleep Med* 2003; **4**: 121–32.

21. International Restless Leg Syndrome Rating Scale. www.medicine.ox.ac.uk/bandolier/booth/RLS/RLSratingscale.pdf (accessed June 2013).

22. Kushida CA, Littner MR, Morgenthaler T, et al. Practice parameters for the indications for polysomnography and related procedures: an update for 2005. *Sleep* 2005; **28**: 499–521.

23. Collop NA, Anderson WM, Boehlecke B, et al. Clinical guidelines for the use of unattended portable monitors in the diagnosis of obstructive sleep apnea in adult patients. Portable Monitoring Task Force of the American Academy of Sleep Medicine. *J Clin Sleep Med* 2007; **3**: 737–47.

24. Collop NA, Tracy SL, Kapur V, et al. Obstructive sleep apnea devices for out-of-center (OOC) testing: technology evaluation. *J Clin Sleep Med* 2011; **7**: 531–48.

25. Littner MR, Kushida C, Wise M, et al. Practice parameters for clinical use of the multiple sleep latency test and the maintenance of wakefulness test. *Sleep* 2005; **28**: 113–21.

26. Sullivan SS, Kushida CA. Multiple sleep latency test and maintenance of wakefulness test. *Chest* 2008; **134**: 854–61.

27. Morgenthaler T, Alessi C, Friedman L, et al. Practice parameters for the use of actigraphy in the assessment of sleep and sleep disorders: an update for 2007. *Sleep* 2007; **30**: 519–29.

28. Girschik J, Fritschi L, Heyworth J, Waters F. Validation of self-reported sleep against actigraphy. *J Epidemiol* 2012; **22**: 462–8.

29. Michaud M, Poirier G, Lavigne G, Montplaisir J. Restless legs syndrome: scoring criteria for leg movements recorded during the suggested immobilization test. *Sleep Med* 2001; **2**: 317–21.

30. Montplaisir J, Boucher S, Nicolas A, et al. Immobilization tests and periodic leg movements in sleep for the diagnosis of restless leg syndrome. *Mov Disord* 1998; **13**: 324–9.

31. Haba-Rubio J, Sforza E. Test-to-test variability in motor activity during the suggested immobilization test in restless legs patients. *Sleep Med* 2006; **7**: 561–6.

Appendix 1 Sleep diary (http://yoursleep.aasmnet.org/pdf/sleepdiary.pdf)

TWO WEEK SLEEP DIARY

INSTRUCTIONS:
1. Write the date, day of the week, and type of day: Work, School, Day Off, or Vacation.
2. Put the letter "C" in the box when you have coffee, cola or tea. Put "M" when you take any medicine.
   Put "A" when you drink alcohol. Put "E" when you exercise.
3. Put a line (I) to show when you go to bed. Shade in the box that shows when you think you fell asleep.
4. Shade in all the boxes that show when you are asleep at night or when you take a nap during the day.
5. Leave boxes unshaded to show when you wake up at night and when you are awake during the day.

SAMPLE ENTRY BELOW: On a Monday when I worked, I jogged on my lunch break at 1 PM, had a glass of wine with dinner at 6 PM, fell asleep watching TV from 7 to 8 PM, went to bed at 10:30 PM, fell asleep around Midnight, woke up and couldn't got back to sleep at about 4 AM, went back to sleep from 5 to 7 AM, and had coffee and medicine at 7:00 in the morning.

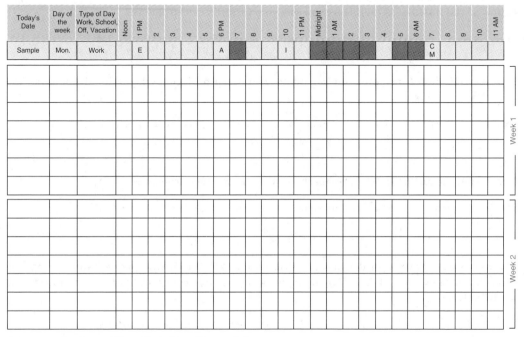

Appendix 2 Stanford Sleepiness Scale (www.stanford.edu/~dement/sss.html)

Degree of sleepiness	Scale rating
Feeling active, vital, alert, or wide awake	1
Functioning at high levels, but not at peak; able to concentrate	2
Awake, but relaxed; responsive but not fully alert	3
Somewhat foggy, let down	4
Foggy; losing interest in remaining awake; slowed down	5
Sleepy, woozy, fighting sleep; prefer to lie down	6
No longer fighting sleep, sleep onset soon; having dream-like thoughts	7
Asleep	X

Data from: Hoddes E, Zarcone V, Smythe H et al. Quantification of sleepiness: a new approach. *Psychophysiology* 1973; 10: 431–6.

Appendix 3 Insomnia Severity Index (ISI) (www.myhealth.va.gov/mhv-portal-web/resources/jsp/help.jsp?helpDirectRequest=sleep_insomnia_indexprint.htm)

Please rate the *CURRENT (i.e. LAST 2 WEEKS) SEVERITY* of your insomnia problem(s).

Insomnia problem	None	Mild	Moderate	Severe	Very severe
1. Difficulty falling asleep	0	1	2	3	4
2. Difficulty staying asleep	0	1	2	3	4
3. Problem waking up too early	0	1	2	3	4

4. How SATISFIED/DISSATISFIED are you with your CURRENT sleep pattern?

Very satisfied	Satisfied	Moderately satisfied	Dissatisfied	Very dissatisfied
0	1	2	3	4

5. How NOTICEABLE to others do you think your sleep problem is in terms of impairing the quality of your life?

Not at all noticeable	A little	Somewhat	Much	Very much noticeable
0	1	2	3	4

6. How WORRIED/DISTRESSED are you about your current sleep problem?

Not at all worried	A little	Somewhat	Much	Very much worried
0	1	2	3	4

7. To what extent do you consider your sleep problem to INTERFERE with your daily functioning (e.g. daytime fatigue, mood, ability to function at work/daily chores, concentration, memory, mood, etc.) CURRENTLY?

Not at all interfering	A little	Somewhat	Much	Very much interfering
0	1	2	3	4

Guidelines for scoring/interpretation

Add the scores for all seven responses.

Total score categories:

0–7	No clinically significant insomnia
8–14	Subthreshold insomnia
15–21	Clinical insomnia (moderate severity)
22–28	Clinical insomnia (severe)

4

Approach to a Patient with Excessive Daytime Sleepiness

Rajdeep Singh, MD[1] and Aatif M. Husain, MD[2,3]

[1] Department of Neurology, Carolinas Medical Center, UNC Chapel Hill, USA
[2] Department of Medicine (Neurology), Duke University Medical Center, USA
[3] Neurodiagnostic Center, Veterans Affairs Medical Center, USA

Introduction

Excessive daytime sleepiness (EDS) refers to an increased likelihood of falling asleep during undesired times. This is often called sleepiness and is a common patient complaint. It is usually ill defined and sometimes loosely associated and merged with symptoms of fatigue and tiredness. EDS as a symptom can lead to impaired quality of life and increased risk of motor vehicle and work-related accidents. Evaluation of a patient with EDS starts with careful history taking followed by a thorough examination. Several ancillary tests are available to help confirm or reject suspicions raised during history and examination.

There are many etiologies of EDS. They range from behaviorally induced causes such as insufficient sleep to serious disorders such as obstructive sleep apnea and narcolepsy. The differential diagnosis of EDS is presented in Box 4.1, and details of these conditions can be found elsewhere in this text.

History

The most important diagnostic method in sleep medicine is skillful history taking. It starts with careful elicitation of the 24-hours sleep-wake cycle with the aim of quantifying sleepiness and its effect on the patient's life. The effect of various other disorders, including pulmonary, cardiac, neurological and psychiatric, affecting sleep should be determined.

> ### Box 4.1 Common causes of excessive daytime sleepiness
>
> Insufficient sleep (behavioral sleep restriction)
> Co-morbid problems (head trauma, stroke, cancer, infections, neurodegenerative conditions)
> Medications
> Psychiatric conditions, especially depression
> Impaired sleep quality:
>
> - Obstructive sleep apnea (OSA)
> - Periodic limb movements of sleep
>
> Primary hypersomnias:
>
> - Narcolepsy
> - Idiopathic hypersomnia
> - Other rare primary hypersomnias including Klein–Levin syndrome

Medications should be reviewed as they can greatly affect sleepiness. The components of a complete sleep history are presented in Box 4.2.

Determining and measuring sleepiness

Sleepiness specifically refers to the likelihood of falling asleep and encompasses decreased alertness, while fatigue and tiredness are associated with difficulty maintaining a high level of performance.[1]

Sleep Medicine in Neurology, First Edition. Edited by Douglas B. Kirsch.
© 2014 John Wiley & Sons, Ltd. Published 2014 by John Wiley & Sons, Ltd.

Sleepiness is considered excessive when it occurs during periods of required alertness. It interferes with occupational and other activities of daily living such as reading, driving, and interacting with others. Every patient with a complaint of sleepiness must be questioned about sleepiness while driving (see Caution box). The occurrence of symptoms during periods of occupation, rest, leisure, work days, weekends or vacations can be an important indicator for differentiating between fatigue and sleepiness.

CAUTION

Sleepiness and driving are a dangerous combination. Sleepiness impairs reaction time, judgment, and vision. The National Transportation Safety Board (NTSB) data suggest that 52% of single motor vehicle accidents were due to fatigue, and sleepiness contributes to up to 100,000 motor vehicle accidents causing about 1500 deaths annually.

In general, estimating sleepiness by the patient's own report is unreliable. Individuals usually underestimate their sleepiness so an observer history should be obtained if possible. The individual patient's motivations and occupational and subjective needs should be kept in mind.

Different scales and questionnaires can be utilized to measure sleepiness and understand its impact on daily life. The most common scale used in clinical practice is the Epworth Sleepiness Scale (ESS) (Box 4.3).[2] This is a self-administered scale used to measure an individual's likelihood of falling asleep in eight different situations. Higher scores mean greater sleepiness. A score less than 10 is normal (no significant sleepiness). The Stanford Sleepiness Scale (SSS) can be used to quantify the

level of sleepiness versus alertness (Table 4.1).[3] This is also a self-rating scale that can be used to rate different time periods or situations. During periods when maximum alertness is needed and expected, the score should be 1. The difference between these two scales is that the ESS measures sleepiness over a longer retrospective time frame (the recent past), whereas the SSS is an assessment of the immediate time period, which may change over the course of any given day. A third scale, the Functional Outcome of Sleep Questionnaire (FOSQ), can be used to assess the impact of excessive sleepiness on functional status. It assesses five domains of everyday living: activity level, vigilance, intimacy, general productivity, and social outcome.

Overview of a typical night's sleep and daytime activity

To understand the patient's sleep quality and sleep hygiene, a structured interview is very helpful. In most cases, history from the bed partner or an observer familiar with the patient's sleep can be very useful in corroborating symptoms or eliciting new ones of which the patient is unaware. Sleep logs and actigraphy (discussed below) can be used in some cases where the history is not clear or when sleep deprivation is suspected as one of the causes of EDS. These tools can also be helpful when a clear schedule is not forthcoming, for patients working rotating shifts and to identify poor sleep hygiene. The key questions that should be asked about nighttime sleep are presented in Box 4.4.

TIPS AND TRICKS

The most common reason for excessive daytime sleepiness is insufficient sleep. This is particularly common among adolescent and young adults. According to a poll conducted by the National Sleep Foundation, 16% of those surveyed slept less than 6 hours on a weekday night.

Daytime naps

Every patient who complains of EDS should be questioned about daytime naps. Unintentional naps during periods of activity such as while working on a computer, in a meeting or lecture, or while talking with others signify significant sleepiness. Intentional

Score chance of dozing at various situations given based the scale below

0 = no chance of dozing
1 = slight chance of dozing
2 = moderate chance of dozing
3 = high chance of dozing

SITUATION   CHANCE OF DOZING

Sitting and reading _____
Watching TV _____
Sitting inactive in a public place (e.g. a theater or a meeting) _____
As a passenger in a car for an hour without a break _____
Lying down to rest in the afternoon when circumstances permit _____
Sitting and talking to someone _____
Sitting quietly after a lunch without alcohol _____
In a car, while stopped for a few minutes in traffic _____

From Hoddes E, Zarcone V, Smythe H, Phillips R, Dement WC. Quantification of sleepiness: a new approach. *Psychophysiology* 1973; **10**: 431–6.

Table 4.1 Stanford Sleepiness Scale. In the SSS the patient is asked to rate their degree of sleepiness during various times of the day or in different situations. This assesses sleepiness at a particular instant in time

Degree of sleepiness	Scale rating
Feeling active, vital, alert or wide awake	1
Functioning at high levels, but not at peak; able to concentrate	2
Awake but relaxed; responsive but not fully alert	3
Somewhat foggy, let down	4
Foggy; losing interest in remaining awake; slowed down	5
Sleepy, woozy, fighting sleep; prefer to lie down	6
No longer fighting sleep, sleep onset soon; having dream-like thoughts	7
Asleep	X

Data from Hoddes E, Zarcone V, Smythe H, Phillips R, Dement WC. Quantification of sleepiness: a new approach. *Psychophysiology* 1973; **10**: 431–6.

Box 4.4 History questions for nighttime sleep

1. What is a typical bedtime schedule? Does it change on weekends or vacations?
2. Do you snore? Has someone refused to sleep in the same room with you or complained about their sleep due to your snoring?
3. Has anyone become worried that you stop breathing during sleep?
4. Have you snorted yourself awake at night?
5. How often do you wake up at night? What are the potential causes of multiple awakenings from the patient's perspective at night? Is it easy to go back to sleep after awakenings?
6. Are your dreams vivid/realistic? Are there vivid dreams as you are falling asleep?
7. How do you feel when you get up in the morning?
8. Do you have frequent morning headaches?
9. Have you ever felt immobile/paralyzed as you are waking up in the morning or while falling asleep?

> ### Box 4.5 History questions for daytime naps
>
> 1. How many naps do you take in a typical day?
> 2. Are your naps intentional or unintentional?
> 3. What times of the day do your naps typically occur? During the morning hours? After lunch?
> 4. How long are your naps?
> 5. How do you feel after your naps? Refreshed?
> 6. Do you dream during your naps? Are the dreams vivid/realistic?
> 7. Have you ever felt immobile/paralyzed when you wake up from a nap?
> 8. Do you have any abnormal movements or behaviors that have been reported to you during naps?
> 9. If you wear a CPAP machine at night, do you wear it during your naps?

napping should also be determined, and that also may suggest excessive sleepiness. Timing of naps should be noted, as those occurring during times of normal circadian dip (early afternoon) may not be as significant as those occurring during times typical of maximal alertness. Duration of naps and how refreshed the patient feels afterwards should be determined. Short naps that refresh the individual are more likely to occur with disorders such as narcolepsy, whereas longer, non-restorative naps are more likely with sleep-disordered breathing (SDB). Patients should be questioned about whether they have vivid dreams or hallucinations during brief naps. Vivid dreams during naps suggest that they are entering rapid eye movement (REM) sleep during their short nap. This is suggestive of REM dysregulation as normally REM sleep first occurs after 90 min of sleep onset. The important questions that should be asked about daytime naps are presented in Box 4.5.

Co-morbid conditions

Various co-morbid conditions can affect overnight sleep, leading to excessive daytime sleepiness and exacerbating primary sleep disorders. During history taking, an attempt should be made to distinguish between EDS caused by co-morbid illnesses

and primary sleep disorders. The common diseases affecting sleep are discussed below.

Pulmonary diseases

Many pulmonary conditions have deleterious effects on oxygenation in sleep. Patients with chronic obstructive pulmonary disease (COPD) have worsening hypoxemia and hypercapnia during sleep. These, along with pulmonary vasoconstriction, predispose patients to the development of pulmonary hypertension and cor pulmonale. Asthma and other allergic conditions, including allergic rhinitis, can cause airway inflammation and constriction. All these conditions can exacerbate SDB. Sleep problems have also been well documented in intrinsic restrictive diseases of the lungs. Questions to screen for these diseases are an important part of the sleep history.

Cardiovascular diseases

There is a consequential and causal relationship between SDB and various cardiovascular disorders. Central sleep apnea (CSA) may be a consequence of congestive heart failure. Hypertension, atrial fibrillation, and coronary artery disease have complex relationships with SDB. The clinical signs and symptoms of SDB in a patient with cardiovascular diseases are often non-specific and diagnosis requires a high index of suspicion in a person complaining of nocturnal dyspnea, chest pain, and palpitations. It is important to ask about snoring and apneic episodes to screen for sleep apnea in these patients. This should particularly be considered in patients with resistant hypertension, intractable heart failure, and recurrent atrial fibrillation.

Neurological diseases

The relationship between sleep disorders and various neurodegenerative disorders is still being defined. Patients with neurological diseases in general seem to have a greater prevalence of sleep disturbance than healthy individuals. Patients with SDB may present with symptoms of cognitive difficulty and memory problems. Epilepsy patients have a higher incidence of hypersomnolence that is often attributed to their medications. However, patients with epilepsy have been found to have greater sleep fragmentation and higher incidence of SDB than the general population. There are also concerns regarding sleep apnea provoking seizures or unmasking an underlying potential for seizures.[4]

Psychiatric diseases

Patients can interpret depression and low energy levels as excessive sleepiness. It can also lead to sleep disruption and poor quality of sleep at night. A low score on the ESS and high score on depression scales such as the Beck Depression Inventory can cue the physician to further exploration of mood disorders.

Other medical conditions

Medical conditions such as chronic pain syndrome, fibromyalgia, gastroesophageal reflux, and genito-urinary diseases can cause sleep disruption, leading to excessive daytime sleepiness. Thyroid problems and liver diseases can also affect sleep.

Medications

Most medications crossing the blood–brain barrier have an effect on sleep architecture and can cause daytime sleepiness. Evaluation of patients with sleep problems is not complete without a review of their medications. This becomes more challenging when a patient has a medical condition that can affect sleep and is taking medications for that condition which can also affect sleep. An example of this may be when a patient with a chronic pain syndrome is taking various analgesic and narcotic medications. The pain syndrome can fragment nocturnal sleep, and the pain medications can cause EDS. Common medication classes that cause EDS are presented in Box 4.6.

Disease-specific questions

Some primary sleep disorders causing hypersomnolence require the elicitation of specific symptoms that might not be covered during the general questions discussed above. For example, reporting symptoms of muscular weakness or loss of muscle control can be suggestive of cataplexy in patients suspected of narcolepsy. Questions specific to primary sleep disorders that can cause EDS are presented in Table 4.2.

Physical examination

Sleep disorders can involve multiple organ systems, requiring sleep physicians to be familiar with the examination of multiple systems. There is no single standard approach; rather, the focus of the examination depends on the differential diagnosis generated during the history.

Box 4.6 Common medications groups that can cause EDS

Sedative hypnotics

- Barbiturates
- Benzodiazepines
- Non-benzodiazepine hypnotics
- Ethanol

Antihypertensives

- Beta-blockers
- Other antihypertensives (methyldopa)

Antidepressants
Antipsychotics
Antihistamines
Anxiolytics
Narcotics
Muscle relaxants
Antiepileptics

Often the physical exam produces limited findings in patients with excessive daytime sleepiness.

General physical examination

The patient's height and weight should be measured and the Body Mass Index calculated. Obstructive sleep apnea is much more common in people with BMI >35. Neck circumference is an important measurement for those suspected of having SDB. Patients with a wide and short neck are especially prone to developing SDB. Check for signs of peripheral arterial disease or varicose veins that can predispose to restless legs syndrome (RLS).

★ TIPS AND TRICKS

Men with neck circumference greater than 17 inches and women with circumference greater than 16 inches are more prone to SDB. Men can be asked for the collar size of their shirt.

Nasal and oropharyngeal examination

Upper airway obstruction is sometimes readily visible during bedside examination. The nose should be examined for patency, polyps, and septal deviation. Oropharyngeal examination should be

Table 4.2 Questions to ask for common primary sleep disorders

Disease name	Specific questions
Narcolepsy	Have you ever felt immobile or paralyzed while falling asleep or in the morning when you are trying to wake up? (Sleep paralysis)
	Have you ever done activities in a semi-automatic fashion without clear memory or consciousness, such as continue to write sentences on the computer that turned out to be nonsensical or continued driving to an unknown location without clear memory of having done so? (Automatic behavior)
	Have you ever had vivid dreams or hallucinations at the time of sleep onset or during short naps? (Hypnogogic hallucinations)
	Have you ever had episodes of muscle weakness during emotional situations such as laughter? (Cataplexy)
	How do you feel after a short nap during the daytime?
Restless legs syndrome	Do you have unpleasant sensations that begin or worsen during periods of inactivity?
	Are these sensations relieved by movement?
	Do these sensations tend to occur or become worse during any particular time period?
	Do these sensations prevent you from going to sleep?
	Has your bed partner or an observer reported frequent movements of your legs during sleep?
Sleep apnea	Do you snore loudly?
	Have you snorted yourself awake at night?
	Has anyone witnessed that you stop breathing at night?
	How do you feel when you get up in the morning?
	Do you have early morning headaches?
	How often do you get up to urinate at night?
Circadian rhythm sleep disorders	What is your sleep-wake schedule?
	What is your bedtime?
	How long does it take to fall asleep?
	What is the most alert period?
	If you were able to create an ideal sleep schedule, what would it be?
	Do you do shift work?
	Is there frequent travel across time zones?

conducted, looking for any abnormalities of facial and jaw structure, tonsillar size and appearance of uvula, soft palate, and tongue. A large tongue base relative to the lateral and anteroposterior diameter of the oropharynx can contribute to upper airway constriction. The Mallampati classification for upper airway patency was originally used by anesthesiologists to assess the difficulty of intubations. It is a rough estimate of the tongue size relative to the oral cavity. The classification provides a score of 1–4, 4 being consistent with severe upper airway constriction. It is based on the anatomical features of the airway seen when the patient opens their mouth and protrudes the tongue (see Figure 2.1, Chapter 2). It provides an independent risk factor for SDB.[5]

★ TIPS AND TRICKS

A common cause of obstructive sleep apnea in thin individuals is retrognathia, a condition in which the mandible or in some cases maxilla is set behind the other at a greater distance than normal. It can be easily evaluated by looking at the neutrally positioned head from the side and comparing the position of the chin relative to the nasion. If the chin lies behind a straight line drawn from the nasion, this indicates retrognathia. Sometimes men grow a beard in an effort make a small mandible more prominent.

Table 4.3 Blood tests to be considered in primary sleep disorders

Test	Indication
Ferritin levels	Restless legs syndrome Used to evaluate secondary cause for restless legs syndrome
Dim light melatonin onset (DLMO)	Circadian rhythm disorders This test measures the onset of melatonin secretion in plasma or saliva
Hypocretin	Narcolepsy. Cerebrospinal fluid hypocretin can be measured in patients suspected of narcolepsy with cataplexy. It is about 90% sensitive and very specific for patients with cataplexy. It can be useful in diagnosis of patients taking REM-suppressant medication that interferes with MSLT results. This test is not very sensitive in narcolepsy patients without cataplexy
HLA DQB1*0602	Narcolepsy. Sensitive for narcolepsy with cataplexy but has low specificity as it is present in about 20% of the general population; low sensitivity for narcolepsy without cataplexy

Cardiopulmonary examination

Pulmonary examination is necessary if SDB is suspected. Cardiovascular examination should be conducted to look for signs of heart failure and pulmonary hypertension. Congestive heart failure is an important cause of central sleep apnea.

Neurological examination

Neurological examination is important for patients with suspected central sleep apnea and various parasomnias. Cranial nerve examination is done to look for brainstem abnormalities that can cause apneas. Parasomnias may be associated with neurodegenerative diseases such as Parkinson's disease, and a motor examination with emphasis on tremor, rigidity, and bradykinesia should be done. Peripheral neuropathy can lead to RLS and should be checked during the sensory examination.

Psychiatric examination

Various psychiatric conditions, including mood disorders, can mimic the hypersomnolence of narcolepsy. Many sleep disorders can co-exist with psychiatric disorders. It is important to evaluate patients' mental status, affect, and motivation.

Investigations and diagnostic tests

The laboratory evaluation of hypersomnolence involves blood tests to rule out any underlying medical condition and specific tests for sleep disorders. The commonly ordered general blood tests include complete blood count (CBC), comprehensive metabolic panel (CMP), and thyroid function panel. Some more specific tests used to evaluate a particular sleep disorder are listed in Table 4.3. Except for ferritin levels in patients suspected of RLS, these tests are not routinely used in clinical practice.

Polysomnogram

A polysomnogram (PSG), also known as a sleep study, involves recording of multiple physiological parameters as the patient sleeps in the sleep laboratory. The common variables recorded in a PSG are shown in Table 4.4.

Table 4.4 Variables recorded during polysomnography

Parameter recorded	Number of channels	Utility
EEG	2–6	Sleep staging
EOG	2	Sleep staging
EMG	3	Sleep staging and record movements
Airflow	1–2	Record airflow
Respiratory belts	2	Measure respiratory effort
Microphone	1	Record snoring
ECG	1	Monitor heart rate and rhythm
Pulse oximetry	1	Monitor oxygen saturation

ECG, electrocardiogram; EEG, electroencephalogram; EMG, electromyogram; EOG, electro-oculogram.

A PSG is most commonly used to evaluate for SDB, though its sensitivity has not been fully studied. It can also be useful for evaluation of suspected periodic limb movements of sleep and parasomnias. Rigorous criteria are used for scoring the PSG. A summary of the PSG is known as the hypnogram. This graphically shows sleep stages, body position, oxygen saturation, heart rate and frequency of arousals, apneas, and leg movements. An example of a hypnogram is shown in Figure 4.1, demonstrating a split night study. The first half of the study was performed for diagnostic purposes and the second part was used for treatment with positive airway pressure (PAP) therapy.

Multiple Sleep Latency Test

The Multiple Sleep Latency Test (MSLT) was originally developed to assess patients with narcolepsy, but has been adapted to objectively measure a patient's level of sleepiness from any cause. It is a daytime test that should be performed after an overnight PSG, which ensures that the patient obtained adequate sleep the night prior to the MSLT. The patient takes 4–5 naps after adequate overnight sleep (deemed as at least 6 hours). The patient is allowed to lie in bed for 20 min in each nap; if they fall asleep, they are allowed to sleep for 15 min. Each nap is separated by a 2-hours interval. The latency to the first stage of sleep is determined for all naps; the average of all latencies is the mean sleep latency. Whether the patient goes into REM sleep in any of the naps is also determined. If REM sleep is present, it is referred to as sleep-onset REM (SOREM). For each MSLT, the mean sleep latency (in minutes) and number of SOREM are reported.

This test is most often done to assess EDS and determine if a patient has narcolepsy. A mean sleep latency of less than 8 min is diagnostic of hypersomnolence. If SOREM is seen in at least two naps along with a mean sleep latency of less than 8 min, it is considered diagnostic of narcolepsy in the correct clinical context.

patient's clinical history. The other possible causes of positive MSLT include insufficient sleep, circadian rhythm disorders, medications, and sleep-disordered breathing. SOREM might be absent in narcolepsy patients taking REM-suppressant medications such as antidepressants.

Maintenance of Wakefulness Test

The Maintenance of Wakefulness Test (MWT) is used to measure daytime alertness and is an indicator of the ability to function and remain alert during periods of inactivity. The patient is asked to stay awake in a sleep-inducing environment. Four such trials of 20 or 40 min are performed with 2-hours intervals between them. The patient is told to refrain from caffeine and other stimulants before or during the time of the test. They are asked not to lie in bed but to sit in a comfortable chair. The patient is not allowed to read or engage in other stimulating activity. The mean sleep onset latency is calculated for all the trials. If the patient falls asleep during the trial, the trial can be terminated before the 20 or 40 min is complete. As such, SOREM are not sought for in an MWT.

There is significant variability among sleep laboratories regarding what is considered a "normal" value of the test. According to the published normative data based on 64 healthy subjects, the mean sleep latency to the first epoch of sustained sleep was 35.2 ± 7.9 min. The lower normal limit, defined as two standard deviations below the mean, was 19.4 min.[4]

The Maintenance of Wakefulness Test has been used to test the effectiveness of stimulants or other treatments on daytime sleepiness. However, it is used most often by regulatory agencies to determine if a patient is alert enough for a particular profession. For example, motor vehicle agencies often require truck drivers to demonstrate their ability to stay awake by undergoing a MWT.

> ✋ **CAUTION**
>
> Though MSLT is commonly used for diagnosis of narcolepsy, its sensitivity and specificity for this condition are limited. It cannot be relied on to "make the diagnosis of narcolepsy" and should always be interpreted within the

> ✋ **CAUTION**
>
> Even though MWT results are often used by regulatory agencies as a marker of sleepiness behind the wheel, there are very limited data indicating that MWT results are predictive of motor vehicle accidents.

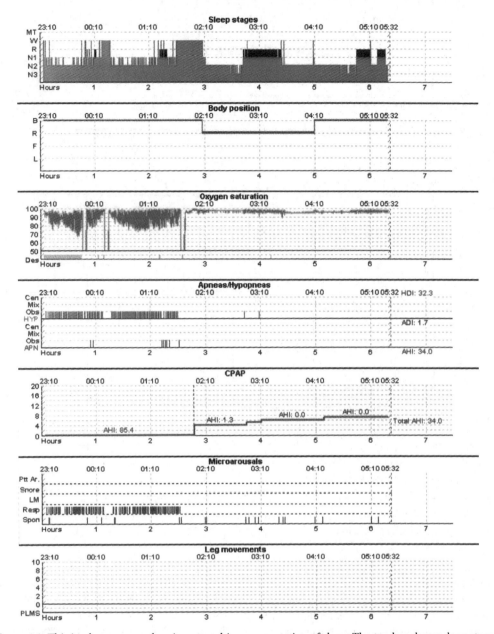

Figure 4.1 This is a hypnogram showing a graphic representation of sleep. The top bar shows sleep stages, including W (wake), R (REM), N1 (stage 1), N2 (stage 2), N3 (stage 3), and MT (movement time). The next bar is position, including B (back), R (right), F (front), and L (left). The third bar is oxygen saturation; notice the frequent desaturations in the first 2.5 hours of sleep that resolve thereafter (after application of CPAP). The next bar shows sleep-disordered breathing (apnea and hypopneas – obstructive, central, and mixed). The fifth bar shows the CPAP pressure used. In the first 2.5 hours of the tracing, CPAP was not used; thereafter, gradually increasing CPAP pressures were used. The next bar shows the arousals, which can be spontaneous or related to respirations, leg movements or snoring. The last bar shows leg movements, which were absent in this example. The hypnogram allows a graphic review of the entire PSG. In this example, the patient had severe obstructive sleep apnea and had very frequent obstructive hypopneas associated with desaturations and arousals (bars 4, 3 and 6, respectively). About 2.5 hours into the study, the patient was put on CPAP (bar 5), and with gradually increasing CPAP pressure, the hypopneas, desaturations, and arousals resolve.

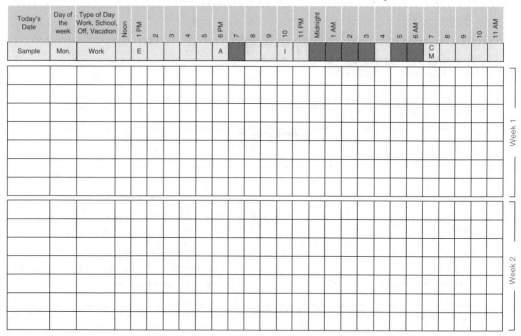

Figure 4.2 Sleep logs are kept for 1–2 weeks and detail many features of sleep during this time. They provide a graphic summary of the patient's self-reported sleep characteristics. ©American Academy of Sleep Medicine, with permission.

Sleep logs

A sleep log is a tool commonly used to supplement a patient's history. It consists of a chart filled out by the patient for a 2–4-week period. It can provide a visual tool to the physician for assessing areas of concern. Sleep logs can be invaluable in identifying patients with behavioral sleep restriction and while treating patients with insomnia and circadian rhythm disorders. However, since it is a self-reported tool, it is subject to social and recall bias. A sample sleep diary provided by the American Academy of Sleep Medicine for patients is shown in Figure 4.2.

Actigraphy

Sleep actigraphs are motion sensors shaped like small watches that are worn by patients usually on the non-dominant wrist. They record movement, which is then used to determine if the patient is awake (movement) or asleep (no movement). Actigraphy is usually recorded for a week at a time and is helpful in defining the patient's sleep-wake schedule. As such, it is most useful in the evaluation of circadian rhythm disorders. Results of actigraphy have been shown to correlate well with measurements of melatonin and core body temperature rhythms.[6] Actigraphy is also helpful in evaluating sleep patterns in patients with insomnia who cannot maintain sleep logs, for studying the effect of treatments designed to improve sleep, shift work sleep disorder and other patients with unusual sleep patterns. An example of an actigraph is presented in Figure 4.3.

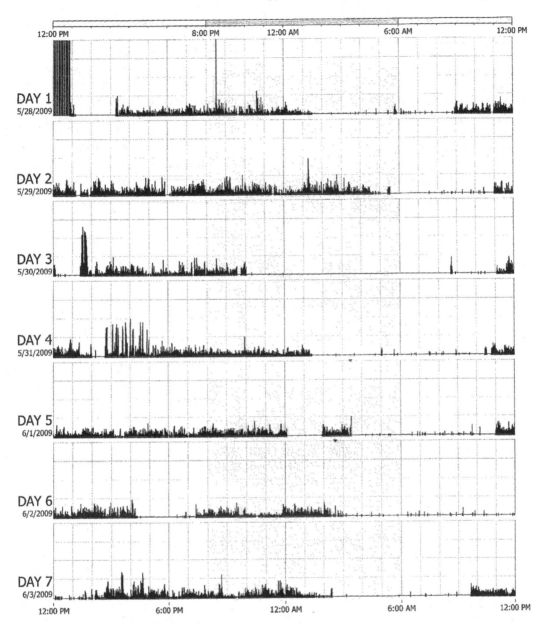

Figure 4.3 In actigraphy, the dark areas indicate movement/activity (wakefulness) and light areas indicate lack of movement/inactivity (sleep). Notice that in this patient the sleep period for Day 1 was from around 1.30 am to 9 am. The other days can be similarly interpreted.

Conclusion

Excessive daytime sleepiness is a common complaint and has many etiologies. It behooves all practitioners to understand the many causes of EDS. An attempt should be made to distinguish between fatigue and EDS. A thorough history and physical examination are very important and are often enough to suggest a diagnosis. Tests specific to sleep disorders, such as the PSG, MSLT, MWT, sleep logs, and actigraphy, provide valuable information and can help confirm a diagnosis suspected on history and examination.

References

1. Carney PR, Berry RB, Geyer JD (eds) *Clinical Sleep Disorders*. Philadelphia: Lippincott Williams and Wilkins, 2005.

2. Johns MW. A new method for measuring daytime sleepiness: the Epworth Sleepiness Scale. *Sleep* 1991; **14**(6): 540–5.

3. Hoddes E, Zarcone V, Smythe H, Phillips R, Dement WC. Quantification of sleepiness: a new approach. *Psychophysiology* 1973; **10**: 431–6.

4. Doghramji K, Mitler MM, Sangal RB, et al. A normative study of the maintenance of wakefulness test (MWT). *Electroencephalogr Clin Neurophysiol* 1997; **103**(5): 554–62.

5. Nuckton TJ, Glidden DV, Browner WS, Claman DM. Physical examination: Mallampati score as an independent predictor of obstructive sleep apnea. *Sleep* 2006; **29**(7): 903–8.

6. Ancoli-Israel S, Cole R, Alessi C, Chambers M, Moorcroft W, Pollak CP. The role of actigraphy in the study of sleep and circadian rhythms. *Sleep* 2003; **26**(3): 342–92.

5

Approach to a Patient with Narcolepsy

Ravichand Madala, MD and Rodney A. Radtke, MD

Department of Neurology, Duke University Medical Center, USA

Introduction

Narcolepsy is one of the most common hypersomnias of central nervous system origin. Its primary symptom is that of excessive daytime sleepiness (EDS). The clinical tetrad of narcolepsy includes EDS, cataplexy, hypnogogic hallucinations, and sleep paralysis.[1] Fragmented nocturnal sleep is often part of the clinical syndrome as well. Sleepiness and cataplexy represent the primary sources of disability of this disorder. Treatment is focused on use of stimulants and other wake-promoting agents to promote alertness. Rapid eye movement (REM)-suppressant medications are used to suppress cataplexy and the other associated auxiliary symptoms of narcolepsy. The recent identification of the loss of hypothalamic hypocretin-containing neurons as the cause of most cases has opened up additional research endeavors to explore how treatment may be more specifically targeted to the underlying pathophysiology of the disorder.

Epidemiology

Narcolepsy is estimated to occur in 0.002–0.18% of the general population. The prevalence is higher in Japanese subjects (0.18%) and lowest in Israeli Jews and Arabs (0.002%).[2] The US prevalence is estimated as between 0.03% and 0.07%, with the condition estimated to occur in 1 in 2000 of Americans.[3] The male-to-female prevalence is equal. The symptoms usually appear in the teens and 20s but in many cases there is a 10-year period between onset and diagnosis. Approximately 50% of adults with the disorder retrospectively report symptoms beginning in their teenage years. Rare cases of onset have been reported in infants and in the elderly.

Clinical symptoms

Excessive sleepiness is often the first reported symptom, followed by cataplexy. Excessive daytime sleepiness alone or in combination with hypnogogic hallucinations and/or sleep paralysis is the presenting symptom in approximately 90% of patients. Using clinical criteria, corresponding to the criteria of the *International Classification of Sleep Disorders*,[1] only 10–15% of patients experience the full tetrad. Approximately 70% of patients have cataplexy, 30% have hypnogogic hallucinations, and 25% have sleep paralysis.[4]

Major symptoms

Excessive sleepiness

The excessive sleepiness seen in narcolepsy is usually characterized by repeated episodes of naps or lapses into sleep of short duration. The typical narcoleptic sleeps for 10–20 min and then awakens refreshed, but with the return of overwhelming sleepiness in the next few hours. Compared to other disorders of excessive sleepiness, the sleepiness is less continually present throughout the day, but episodically becomes overwhelming, leading to what are sometimes described as "sleep attacks." There is no increase in total sleep time per 24 hours, as can be seen in other hypersomnias, such as idiopathic hypersomnia. The excessive sleepiness in narcolepsy often interferes with daytime functioning and work performance. It may also interfere with memory, concentration, and cognitive abilities.

Sleep Medicine in Neurology, First Edition. Edited by Douglas B. Kirsch.
© 2014 John Wiley & Sons, Ltd. Published 2014 by John Wiley & Sons, Ltd.

Cataplexy

This is a sudden decrement in muscle tone leading to muscle weakness, paralysis, or postural collapse. These symptoms are variable in severity, and are often subtle, primarily affecting the knees or face (droopy face, slurring of speech). There is usually bilateral loss of muscle tone. Cataplexy is usually triggered by a sudden emotion such as laughter or anger. Other triggering emotions include embarrassment, sexual arousal, or startle. Some patients may report cataplexy to only specific idiosyncratic stimuli. Episodes generally last for seconds to minutes with a frequency ranging from daily to monthly. The loss of muscle tone is due to the intrusion of the atonia normally seen during REM sleep into wakefulness. The diaphragm and ocular muscles are unaffected. During the episode the patient is awake initially, but can fall asleep if it is a prolonged episode. The patient is aware of the surroundings and can remember details of the event, which differentiate this from other episodic disorders such as epileptic seizures. Cataplexy, when severe, may be the most disabling feature of narcolepsy due to falls and injuries. A rare complication of cataplexy is *status cataplecticus* in which repeated cataplectic attacks last for hours to days. It can occur spontaneously but usually is seen with abrupt discontinuation of REM-suppressant medications.

> ★ TIPS AND TRICKS
>
> During cataplexy, respiration and voluntary eye movements are not compromised. Consciousness is preserved during the episode. On examination, deep tendon reflexes are absent.

Hypnagogic hallucinations

These are vivid sensory images that occur during the transition from wakefulness to sleep. They are particularly vivid with sleep-onset REM periods. They can be visual, auditory, or tactile in nature. They are remarkably real in character, often perceived as threatening to the individual, and difficult for the individual to differentiate from reality. As such, the patient will often act on the hallucinatory content, e.g. run out of the house due to the perception that the house is on fire.

Sleep paralysis

Immobility of the body or inability to speak that occurs in the transition between sleep and wakefulness. Episodes of sleep paralysis are thought to be due to the intrusion of the muscle atonia of REM sleep into wakefulness. These episodes end spontaneously after seconds to minutes, but often can be abruptly terminated with the touch of a bed partner. Patients often report feeling unable to breathe. Initially these events may be quite disturbing but with time they become less concerning unless associated with hallucinatory content. Isolated sleep paralysis, not associated with narcolepsy, varies among ethnic groups and may occur in up to 5–30% of the normal population.[5]

> ★ TIPS AND TRICKS
>
> Isolated sleep paralysis is common, particularly during periods of sleep deprivation or stress. In the absence of any other symptoms of narcolepsy, the patient should be reassured as to the benign nature of the symptom and that no additional testing is likely warranted.

Associated symptoms

Nocturnal sleep disruption usually is not present early on but in well-established narcolepsy, sleep disruption is common. Patients fall asleep readily but wake up every 60–90 min with periods of sustained wakefulness. Also, acting out dreams (REM behavior disorder), vivid dreams, and automatic behaviors (a manifestation of EDS) can be associated with narcolepsy. Automatic behaviors, such as completing a mundane task without remembering it, is commonly seen in patients with severe sleepiness but is not specific for narcolepsy as it can be seen in other disorders such as sleep apnea or severe sleep deprivation.

Pathophysiology

The pathophysiology is unclear. There is some evidence that genetic predisposition, abnormal neurotransmitter functioning, and abnormal immune modulation may all play a role in the development of narcolepsy. HLA DQB1*0602 is positive in 85% of patients with narcolepsy with cataplexy. Loss of hypocretin-1 secreting cells in the hypothalamus secondary to an autoimmune mechanism has been postulated.[6] Hypocretin neurons project onto monoaminergic and cholinergic neurons which are involved in the regulation of sleep. A dysfunction of the central sleep regulation leads to inappropriate transitions between sleep and wake, throughout the entire 24-hours period. In narcolepsy, patients have been shown to have a decreased level of hypocretin in the cerebrospinal fluid. The absence of hypocretin causes an imbalance of the motor excitation and inhibition. Emotional stimuli may precipitate this state, causing inactivation of motor excitation and activation of the inhibitory system.

Differential diagnosis

History is important in evaluating other possible causes of EDS. Diagnostic testing with a polysomnogram and next-day Multiple Sleep Latency Test (MSLT) helps to eliminate other causes of EDS such as sleep apnea, periodic limb movements of sleep, and idiopathic hypersomnia. Narcolepsy can be differentiated from idiopathic hypersomnia by many key features (see Table 5.1). There is an increased incidence of sleep apnea in narcoleptics which complicates the diagnosis.

Diagnosis

The diagnosis can be made by history alone, when the history of EDS is accompanied by definite cataplexy. Cataplexy is essentially pathognomonic of narcolepsy. Even in other disorders where cataplexy is described (multiple sclerosis, Prader–Willi, etc.),

Table 5.1 Differentiating narcolepsy and idiopathic hypersomnia

	Narcolepsy	Idiopathic hypersomnia
Naps restorative?	Usually yes	Usually no
Cataplexy?	Yes	No
REM intrusion?	Yes	No
Disrupted nocturnal sleep?	Usually yes	Usually no
Prolonged sleep need?	Usually no	Usually yes
MSLT results?	MSL <8 min SOREM >=2	MSL <8 min SOREM <2

MSL, mean sleep latency; MSLT, Multiple Sleep Latency Test; SOREM, sleep-onset rapid eye movement.

the cataplexy is not as abrupt and not as consistently associated with emotion. Sleep paralysis and hypnogogic hallucinations, while suggestive of narcolepsy, are seen in the normal population and therefore are less useful in the clinical diagnosis of narcolepsy.

The physical and neurological examination is usually normal and there is really no finding on physical examination that adds to the diagnostic evaluation. An abnormal neurological exam should raise the suspicion of a different etiology and would likely warrant an imaging study of the brain. Of note, if the examiner has a chance to witness an attack of cataplexy, the examination would show a decreased tone in the extremities and a transient loss of deep tendon reflexes.

> ### ✋ CAUTION
>
> Neurological exams in patients with narcolepsy are normal and brain imaging studies are not usually indicated. If neurological exam is abnormal, brain imaging may be warranted to exclude central nervous system (CNS) abnormalities such as multiple sclerosis, stroke, or brainstem tumor that can rarely give rise to narcolepsy.

Several sleepiness scales are available to help assess excessive sleepiness. The most commonly used is the Epworth Sleepiness Scale (ESS). Excessive sleepiness correlates with an ESS score >10. Narcolepsy patients, who in general have a severe degree of sleepiness, have a mean ESS of 18.[7]

The International Classification of Sleep Disorders has recognized four categories of narcolepsy: narcolepsy with cataplexy, narcolepsy without cataplexy, narcolepsy due to a medical condition with or without cataplexy, and unspecified narcolepsy.[1] Narcolepsy due to a medical condition can be due to type C Niemann–Pick disease, Prader–Willi, sarcoidosis, multiple sclerosis, or a lesion in the hypothalamic region. Unspecified narcolepsy is a temporary classification until additional information is obtained for more precise classification.

Laboratory studies

More than 85% of narcoleptics with cataplexy share a specific HLA allele, DQB1*0602.[8] HLA DQBI*0602 is present in 20% of the general population which makes having the HLA alleles of no diagnostic value. In certain clinical situations, it may be helpful to use the assay to exclude or lessen the likelihood of narcolepsy. However, HLA testing is not part of the usual diagnostic evaluation of a patient with possible narcolepsy. Cerebrospinal fluid (CSF) hypocretin levels below 110 pg/mL are strongly supportive of the diagnosis of narcolepsy.[9] In CSF, normal values are >200 pg/mL, with an average around 350 pg/mL.[10] However, it is primarily sensitive in patients in narcolepsy with cataplexy, so its utility is limited since cataplexy is pathognomonic for narcolepsy and the diagnosis can be confidently made from history and sleep laboratory testing. Neurodegenerative, neuromuscular, and immune-mediated diseases, as well as traumatic brain injury, have also been shown to have low CSF hypocretin levels.[10]

Imaging studies

Typically imaging studies are unrevealing and are not usually warranted unless there is a clinical suspicion of a CNS abnormality that may be contributing to the patient's symptoms. A few small studies have shown magnetic resonance imaging (MRI) changes of the pons within the reticular activating system and idiopathic narcolepsy may be due to structural abnormalities of the diencephalon and brainstem.[11]

Polysomnography

An overnight polysomnogram (PSG) followed by a next-day MSLT is the standard work-up in patients with suspected narcolepsy or hypersomnolence. Stimulants should be discontinued 2 weeks prior to the PSG and MSLT to avoid inaccurate results. The overnight polysomnogram will exclude sleep apnea and period limb movements of sleep as causes for disrupted nighttime sleep. The MSLT will provide information about the degree of hypersomnolence and the presence of sleep-onset REM periods (SOREM). The MSLT involves five opportunities to nap at 2-hours intervals during the daytime. Two or more SOREM and a mean sleep latency (MSL) of less than 8 min strongly suggest narcolepsy in the correct clinical context. In previous studies in patients with narcolepsy, the MSL was found to be <3 min.[7] These findings are not completely specific and also can be seen in patients with sleep deprivation and sleep apnea. Also, it is important to note

that the use of stimulant or sedative medications (or their abrupt withdrawal) may affect the results. It is usually recommended that REM-suppressant medication (selective serotonin reuptake inhibitor [SSRI] antidepressants) and stimulant medication be discontinued before undergoing sleep lab evaluation with a MSLT.

Management

A multimodal approach with pharmacological therapy and behavioral therapy is required to treat narcolepsy. The patients should be instructed to:

- maintain a regular sleep schedule, getting adequate sleep at night with good sleep hygiene
- avoid heavy meals, high sugar snacks, and alcohol since these may contribute to "sleep attacks"
- schedule short naps (brief 10–20 min naps) which usually result in improved alertness. Narcolepsy patients should talk to their family, friends, and employers about their disease so they can understand that naps (which are usually restorative) can improve productivity and are not indicative of laziness or lack of interest
- not drive or operate heavy machinery when sleepy
- exercise daily, which can have stimulating effects.

Approach to pharmacotherapy

Effective pharmacotherapy can require multiple medications. Stimulant medications are used to treat excessive sleepiness and REM-suppressant medications are used to treat cataplexy. Sodium oxybate can treat both EDS and cataplexy. Modafinil and armodafinil are chosen as first-line stimulant medications due to their limited side-effect profile. Commonly used older stimulant medications include methylphenidate and dextroamphetamine. Newer REM-suppressant medications that are effective in cataplexy include the antidepressant venlafaxine.

Stimulant medications for excessive sleepiness (see Table 5.2)

- Modafinil (Provigil) is a wake-promoting agent that is thought to alter levels of dopamine, gamma-aminobutyric acid (GABA), or norepinephrine. It has few side-effects with the most

Table 5.2 Medications commonly used for excessive sleepiness

Medication	Action	Half-life (hours)	Dose (mg/day)	Side-effects
Modafinil	Promotes wakefulness	9–14	200–400	Nausea, HA, induces P450 and increases metabolism of oral contraceptives
Armodafinil	Promotes wakefulness	15	150–250	Nausea, HA, induces P450 and increases metabolism of oral contraceptives
Methylphenidate	CNS stimulant	2–7	10–60	Cardiovascular stimulation, drug tolerance, rebound hypersomnolence
Dextroamphetamine	CNS stimulant	10–12	5–60	Cardiovascular stimulation, drug tolerance, rebound hypersomnolence
Sodium oxybate	CNS depressant	0.5–1	4500–9000	Nausea, headache

CNS, central nervous system.

common being headache. Sympathomimetic activation is much lower compared to the traditional stimulants and as such, these agents are associated with much less hypertension and tachycardia. Modafinil's maximum concentration is reached in 2–4 hours. The dose can be taken in a single morning dose or split into a morning dose upon awakening and a noontime or midday dose. Usually the dosage range is 200–400 mg per day, but higher doses may provide additional benefit.

- Armodafinil (Nuvigil) is the r-enantiomer of modafinil and is primarily distinguished by its longer half-life which results in it being given once a day. Its side-effect profile is similar to modafinil. The dosage range is 150–250 mg daily.
- Methylphenidate (Ritalin) is one of the oldest and most frequently used stimulant medications. It is thought to act primarily through brainstem dopamine, nigrostriatal, and mesocorticolimbic pathways. It does not have major effects on monoamine storage and leads to milder side-effects than amphetamines. The side-effects include irritability, headache, nervousness, palpitations, insomnia, dyskinesias, anorexia, nausea, sweating, and psychosis. The dose is 10–60 mg a day divided in 2–3 doses during the daytime. Patients may need additional doses for certain occasions (such as before driving), along with their usual scheduled daily dosages. Sustained-release formulations are

available for methylphenidate (as well as dextroamphetamine) and are often preferred as they avoid frequent doses of the medication and the "crash" that many patients experience as the stimulant medication wears off and the patient feels even more sleepy than before taking the medication.

- Amphetamines: the most commonly used is dextroamphetamine (Dexedrine) which works by releasing dopamine and noradrenaline. Amphetamines have a longer half-life than methylphenidate. The side-effect profile is similar to methylphenidate but the side-effects tend to be more more prominent. The usual dosage range is 5–60 mg daily.

Note: Mazindol is a weak releasing agent of dopamine and has been withdrawn from the market in several countries due to reports of cardiac valvular abnormalities resulting from its use. Selegiline, a monoamine oxidase B (MAO-B), is rarely used due to the need to maintain a low tyramine diet to avoid hypertensive crisis.

⚜ CAUTION

Modafinil and armodafinil induce the P450 system and increase the metabolism of oral contraceptives, amongst other medications. Women using birth control pills should be counseled regarding this issue.

Table 5.3 Medications commonly used for cataplexy

Medication	Mechanism	Half-life (hours)	Dose (mg/day)	Side-effects
Venlafaxine	Serotonin and norepinephrine reuptake inhibitor (SNRI)	5	37.5–300	Gastrointestinal upset
Clomipramine	SNRI	32	10–200	Nausea, anorexia, dry mouth, urinary retention, tachycardia
Sodium oxybate	Gamma-aminobutyric acid	0.5–1	4500–9000	Nausea, headache

Rapid eye movement-suppressant medications for cataplexy (see Table 5.3)

- Venlafaxine (Effexor) is a serotonin and noradrenaline reuptake inhibitor (SNRI). It is an antidepressant with some stimulating effects and should be taken in the morning to avoid nighttime sleep disruption. Its major side-effect is gastrointestinal upset. The dosage range is 37.5–300 mg daily.
- Tricyclic antidepressants (TCAs) have been used to treat cataplexy. The most commonly used medications in this class are clomipramine and protriptyline. Possible mechanisms include anticholinergic effects, adrenergic reuptake inhibition, or serotonergic reuptake inhibition. Clomipramine is typically used at a dose of 25–75 mg daily but lower doses of 10–20 mg are often effective. Protriptyline is used at a dose of 2.5–10 mg daily. The major adverse effects of these tricyclic antidepressants are the anitcholinergic side-effects. Contrary to the slow onset of TCA efficacy in treating depression, the cataplexy-suppressing effects are almost immediately seen upon initiating these drugs, but the effect is not sustained and multiple doses throughout the day are usually needed.
- Selective serotonin reuptake inhibitors (SSRIs) (such as fluoxetine) are sometimes used, but are less effective then the SNRI antidepressent medications.

Note: monoamine oxidase inhibitors (MAOI), while strong REM suppressants, are not commonly used due to numerous side-effects and drug interactions. Atomoxetine (Strattera) is a noradrenergic uptake inhibitor that has been used to decrease cataplexy but there has been rare but potential liver toxicity reported.

Sodium oxybate

Sodium oxybate (Xyrem) is the only treatment for cataplexy which is FDA approved.[12] It is a potent short-acting hypnotic that can be used to treat EDS in narcolepsy.[13] Sodium oxybate is an endogenous metabolite of GABA. It has been shown to decrease nocturnal awakening, increase slow-wave sleep, and consolidates REM sleep. The starting dose is 4.5 g divided in two doses taken at nighttime. The first dose is taken as the patient gets into bed. The nighttime doses are taken 3–4 hours apart and thus typically the patient has to set an alarm to wake them to take the second dose. The doses are increased every 1–2 weeks up to a maximum dosage of 9 g per day. Improvement is noticed within the first 3 months.

Sodium oxybate is usually used in patients with moderate-to-severe symptoms of narcolepsy. It is a CNS depressant medication and alcohol or other CNS depressants must be avoided during its use. Sodium oxybate improves daytime sleepiness, but concomitant use of modafinil or another stimulant medication is usually required. While clearly an effective agent for narcolepsy, some patients discontinue its use due to concerns regarding parasomnias (confusional arousals) or the effects of the heavy salt load present in the medication.

⚠ **CAUTION**

Gamma-hydroxybutyrate (GHB) has been used illegally as a "date rape" drug. Patients who take sodium oxybate, the sodium salt of GHB, should be counseled to take this medication in a safe environment. Due to concern about misuse of the drug, it is available only from a single mail order pharmacy and is sent by overnight delivery directly to the patient.

⚠ CAUTION

Due to insufficient clinical studies, stimulant and anticataplectic drugs are not typically recommended in pregnancy unless absolutely necessary. Most patients discontinue the medications prior to pregnancy. However, sodium oxybate is considered a class B medication for pregnant women.

Prognosis and complications

Patients tend to have a good response to treatment and have improved daytime performance. The excessive sleepiness decreases with stimulant medications. Episodes of cataplexy lessen with sodium oxybate or other REM suppressants. Co-morbid medical problems can develop, including sleep apnea, period limb movements of sleep, REM behavior disorder, depression, eating disorders, and diabetes.[14] Motor vehicle accidents are common and the patient should be counseled about not driving or operating heavy machinery when sleepy.

★ TIPS AND TRICKS

Most states do not have laws governing the operating of motor vehicles while sleepy, so there is no legal restriction of narcoleptic patients with respect to driving. However, individuals with narcolepsy are significantly more likely to be involved in motor vehicle accidents and should be advised to be aware of the potential dangers of driving and restrict driving if necessary.

Future treatments and therapies

The current treatments for narcolepsy are directed at the specific symptoms noted above. With developments in understanding the neurobiological basis of the disease, newer therapies are likely to emerge. Potential new therapies include medications that are histamine agonists to promote wakefulness and histamine antagonists for sedation. Thyrotropin-releasing hormone agonists have alerting properties and have been shown to increase wakefulness and decrease cataplexy in animals. Hypocretin deficiency is thought to be the cause of narcolepsy with cataplexy. Newer therapies are being explored with the aim of replacing this deficient neurotransmitter. These efforts include intranasal hypocretin administration, cell transplantation, and gene therapy. Narcolepsy is presumed to be an autoimmune disorder and therapy with intravenous immunoglobulin or plasmapheresis has been reported and offers a potential area of intervention to avoid or arrest the development of narcolepsy.

References

1. American Academy of Sleep Medicine. *International Classification of Sleep Disorders*, 2nd edn. Westchester, IL: American Academy of Sleep Medicine, 2005.
2. Longstreth WT Jr, Koepsell TD, Ton TG, Hendrickson AF, van Belle G. The epidemiology of narcolepsy. *Sleep* 2007; **30**(1): 13–26.
3. Ohayon MM, Ferini-Strambi L, Plazzi G, et al. Frequency of narcolepsy symptoms and other sleep disorders in narcoleptic patients and their first-degree relatives. *J Sleep Res* 2005; **14**(4): 437–45.
4. Overeem S, Mignot E, van Dijk JG, et al. Narcolepsy: clinical features, new pathological insights, and future perspectives. *J Clin Neurophysiol* 2001; **18**: 78–105.
5. Dahlitz M, Parkes JD. Sleep paralysis. *Lancet* 1993; **341**: 406–7.
6. Black JL 3rd, Silber MH, Krahn LE, et al. Analysis of hypocretin (orexin) antibodies in patients with narcolepsy. *Sleep* 2005; **28**(4): 427–31.
7. Sangal RB, Mitler MM, Sangal JM. Subjective sleepiness ratings (Epworth sleepiness scale) do not reflect the same parameter of sleepiness as objective sleepiness (maintenance of wakefulness test) in patients with narcolepsy. *Clin Neurophysiol* 1999; **110**: 2131–5.
8. Mignot E. Genetic and familial aspects of narcolepsy. *Neurology* 1998; **50**(2 Suppl 1): S16–22.

9. Mignot E, Lammers GJ, Ripley B, et al. The role of cerebrospinal fluid hypocretin measurement in the diagnosis of narcolepsy and other hypersomnias. *Arch Neurol* 2002; **59**(10): 1553–62.

10. Fronczek R, Baumann CR, Lammers GJ, Bassetti CL, Overeem S. Hypocretin/orexin disturbances in neurological disorders. *Sleep Med Rev* 2009; **13**(1): 9–22.

11. Bassetti C, Aldrich MS, Quint DJ. MRI findings in narcolepsy. *Sleep* 1997; **20**(8): 630–1.

12. US Xyrem1 Multicenter Study Group. A 12-month, open-label, multicenter extension trial of orally administered sodium oxybate for the treatment of narcolepsy. *Sleep* 2003; **26**(1): 31–5.

13. Black J, Houghton WC. Sodium oxybate improves excessive daytime sleepiness in narcolepsy. *Sleep* 2006; **29**(7): 939–46.

14. Daniels E, King MA, Smith IE, Shneerson JM. Health-related quality of life in narcolepsy. *J Sleep Res* 2001; **10**(1): 75–81.

6

Evaluation and Medical Management of Sleep-Disordered Breathing

Mihaela H. Bazalakova, MD, PhD[1,2] and Lawrence J. Epstein, MD[1,3]

[1] Division of Sleep Medicine, Department of Medicine, Brigham and Women's Hospital, USA
[2] Department of Neurology, Massachusetts General Hospital, USA
[3] Harvard Medical School, USA

Introduction and epidemiology

Sleep-disordered breathing (SDB) consists of a variety of disorders characterized by respiratory or ventilatory disturbance during sleep. Consequences include excessive daytime sleepiness (EDS), cognitive dysfunction, and cardiovascular disease. There are two primary types: obstructive sleep apnea (OSA), caused by blockage or collapse of the upper airway, and central sleep apnea (CSA), defined by cessation of airflow due to the absence of respiratory effort despite an open airway. SDB is underdiagnosed and undertreated, not only in the general population but in patients with neurological disorders who may be at increased risk. Neurological conditions which may result in or exacerbate pre-existing SDB include motor neuron disorders, congenital or acquired myopathies, diabetic or other neuropathy, neuromuscular junction dysfunction, and a range of vascular, demyelinating or neurodegenerative insults to the cortex or brainstem respiratory centers [1] (see Box 6.2).

Obstructive SDB represents a spectrum from partial to total closure of the airway, and phenotypes reflect the degree of airway closure. Primary snoring is due to mild airway narrowing. Further narrowing of the airway increases airway resistance and can trigger respiratory effort-related arousals (RERAs) and present as snoring and daytime sleepiness, sometimes referred to as the upper airway resistance syndrome (UARS). OSA is defined as airway narrowing that reduces or eliminates airflow and causes a drop in oxyhemoglobin saturation and/or an arousal from sleep.

As OSA is the most commonly encountered SDB disorder, it is better characterized epidemiologically. Studies place the prevalence of moderate-to-severe OSA in the middle-aged population in the 3–5% range. However, it is estimated that 50–75% of patients affected by OSA remain undiagnosed, bringing the actual suspected prevalence as high as 20%, especially in those over 65 years of age. OSA underdiagnosis is likely multifactorial, partially due to unawareness and lack of screening effort on the part of providers, but also because up to 50% of patients, including those with severe OSA, are unaware of or underestimate their own symptoms.

Central sleep apnea is a more heterogeneous disorder with a variety of patterns and etiologies. Cheyne-Stokes respiration, a waxing and waning or periodic breathing pattern, occurs most commonly in congestive heart failure (CHF) patients, occurring in up to 40% of patients with an ejection fraction <40%. A similar pattern is seen in high-altitude periodic breathing and is associated with ascent to higher elevations. Congenital hypoventilation syndromes are rare disorders that result in the absence

Sleep Medicine in Neurology, First Edition. Edited by Douglas B. Kirsch.
© 2014 John Wiley & Sons, Ltd. Published 2014 by John Wiley & Sons, Ltd.

of ventilatory drive and effort during sleep and can be fatal if not recognized quickly. Nervous system injury and opiate effects can also cause hypoventilation or apnea. The approach to CSA is to identify the particular etiology, treat any correctable underlying cause, and provide treatment particular to the CSA type.

Pathogenesis

⚙ SCIENCE REVISITED

Obstructive sleep apnea is commonly exacerbated during rapid eye movement (REM) sleep, secondary to atonia of the oropharyngeal muscles, including the genioglossus. Alcohol and muscle relaxants similarly worsen OSA severity through reduction in resting muscle tone.

Pathophysiology of obstructive sleep apnea

Obstructive sleep apnea is characterized by repetitive complete or partial collapse of the airway during sleep, leading to airflow impedance to varying degrees, and resulting in hypoxemia, hypercapnia, sympathetic surges, and sleep fragmentation. Any factors that predispose to a narrow nasal-oropharynx in turn facilitate airway collapse and, thus, OSA manifestation. Anatomical characteristics that result in a crowded airway include a small bony window at baseline, narrowing of the lateral pharyngeal walls from fat deposition in the soft tissues, an enlarged tongue, a visceral pattern of truncal obesity, and mechanical narrowing of the nasopharynx. All of these result in OSA patients having reduced upper airway size compared to those without OSA. In addition to underlying anatomy or obesity, OSA can result from acquired extra- or intraluminal obstruction, for example nasopharyngeal tumors or vocal cord paralysis. Active tobacco use and hypothyroidism have emerged as risk factors for the development of OSA, the latter likely through the development of macroglossia and impaired on upper airway muscle function.

However, OSA is a primary disorder of sleep, and its basis lies in the differential innervation of the oropharyngeal muscles during sleep, as opposed to the awake state. The pharyngeal dilator muscles stiffen in response to negative intrapharyngeal pressure during inspiration in order to prevent airway collapse, a process known as the upper airway negative pressure reflex. While some muscles, including the genioglossus (GG), show phasic activity, others are tonically active, and this likely reflects differential innervation by motor nuclei controlled by medullary neurons involved in respiratory control. While awake, the upper airway negative pressure reflex compensates for the reduced airway size, maintaining airway patency. During sleep, the negative pressure reflex is decreased, resulting in diminished resting muscle tone, leading to airway narrowing, increased upper airway resistance, and potential for airway compromise.

As a salient illustration of the importance of sleep-dependent physiological determinants of OSA, apnea severity often, although not always, peaks in the REM sleep state, which is characterized by muscle atonia. Additionally, the muscle relaxant properties of alcohol and benzodiazepines are recognized precipitants of OSA exacerbation. Pharyngeal muscle denervation secondary to dysfunction at the neuromuscular junction, or involvement by an underlying myopathy, can be expected to lead to increased susceptibility to SDB in patients with neuromuscular disorders ranging from diabetic neuropathy to motor neuron disease to myasthenia gravis to muscular dystrophy. Electromyographic (EMG) recordings from the GG muscle in OSA patients show prolonged motor unit potentials (MUPs), similar to changes seen in neuropathic denervation, suggesting a compromised neuromuscular reserve in OSA patients. Increasingly sophisticated research into the underlying pathophysiology of OSA continues to elucidate additional factors affecting the development of OSA, including the importance of the arousal threshold, or the variable response to increases in respiratory effort that can be tolerated by the individual without electroencephalogram (EEG) changes consistent with a momentary awakening – another neurologically relevant parameter.

Pathophysiology of central sleep apnea

Similarly to OSA, CSA is characterized by recurrent cessation of airflow, with associated hypoxia, hypercarbia, sympathetic surges, and microarousals. The important difference is that the airway is open and compensatory respiratory effort is absent. Hence the designation of "central" sleep apnea, implying a lack of ventilatory drive from central nervous system neurons of the medullary respiratory centers. Of note, parameters other than failure of brainstem respiratory drive may lead to the same polysomnographic pattern. For example, a myopathy or complete breakdown at the diaphragmatic or pharyngeal dilator neuromuscular junctions can cause a decrease in airflow and lack of measurable chest or abdominal expansion. In these cases, the designation of "central" apnea may be counterintuitive to the neurologist, as the failure is postsynaptic. CSA may result from acquired insults to the brainstem respiratory centers, including vascular or demyelinating disorders such as medullary stroke or multiple sclerosis, space-occupying lesions such as primary or metastatic brainstem tumors, or pharmacologically induced respiratory depression secondary to opiate use. CSA can also be seen in congenital syndromes, such as congenital central hypoventilation syndrome (CCHS) or Ondine's curse, characterized by hypoventilation during sleep or, in more severe cases, even during the awake state. Additional manifestations of autonomic dysfunction can be seen in cases of CCHS including agenesis of myenteric postganglionic neurons or Hirschsprung's disease.

Central sleep apnea is commonly seen in CHF where it manifests as the Cheyne-Stokes respiration (CSR) pattern. CSR can be characterized as a ventilatory instability or "high loop gain" problem, where patients hypo- and hyperventilate out of proportion to changes in $PaCO_2$ levels. The typical response to sleep onset is a decrease in ventilation and a slight increase in $PaCO_2$. In patients with CSR, rising $PaCO_2$ levels lead to exaggerated hyperventilation which overshoots the $PaCO_2$ set point and leads to hypocapnia, hypoventilation, and apnea. This again triggers hyperventilation, starting the cycle of crescendo-decrescendo breathing.

Circulatory delay is one mechanism hypothesized to underlie CSR in CHF; another proposed etiology is a centrally mediated abnormal response to changing $PaCO_2$ levels. CSA with CSR also occurs in renal failure, with altered $PaCO_2$ chemosensitization, and at high altitudes.

Treatment-emergent central sleep apnea

In a certain subset of patients, positive airway pressure (PAP) treatment of OSA exacerbates preexisting or unmasks new CSA. This pattern, sometimes called complex sleep apnea, is often more prominent in non-REM (NREM) sleep and, in contrast to OSA, improves during REM sleep. It is frequently characterized by modest oxygen desaturations and hypocarbia, and often consists of shorter crescendo-decrescendo respiratory cycles, typically 30 sec in duration, compared to >45 sec seen in CSR-CSA. Predictors of complex sleep apnea include co-morbid CHF or opiate use, severe OSA, central apnea index (CAI) >5/hour or CSR on PAP, and >50% of baseline apnea hypopnea index (AHI) composed of central rather than obstructive apneas.

In summary, SDB comprises a group of disorders with a variety of causal mechanisms that result in a common endpoint of sleep-induced respiratory compromise. Where an individual patient stands within this group appears to be determined by a combination of their unique anatomical, neuromuscular, and neurophysiological characteristics. Current research is focused on developing individualized therapy tailored to the specific underlying pathophysiology, thus improving compliance and outcomes.

Postulated mechanisms of sleep-disordered breathing's effect on end-organ systems

Large population-based studies, as well as smaller prospective cohort studies, have provided cross-sectional and observational data linking moderate and severe OSA with refractory hypertension, increased risk of ischemic heart disease, stroke,[2] atrial fibrillation, insulin resistance, and increased mortality associated with cardio- and cerebrovascular disease.[3] A number of mechanisms contribute to the relationship between OSA and the range of related medical conditions.

Intermittent hypoxia and reoxygenation

With the presumed associated oxidative damage, these constitute the most commonly proposed mechanism of end-organ tissue damage in OSA. Upregulation of reactive oxygen species and downstream proinflammatory cytokines, including tumor necrosis factor alpha (TNF-alpha), interleukin 6 (IL-6), and C-reactive protein (CRP), have been implicated in premature atherosclerosis and endothelial dysfunction, leading to long-term cardio- and cerebrovascular consequences in OSA patients. Dysregulation of angiotensin II and endothelin has been implicated in hypoxia-induced vascular remodeling.

Sympathetic nervous system overactivation

This has been demonstrated both as acute surges in muscle sympathetic nerve activity (MSNA) following apneas and hypopneas, and as a chronic consequence of OSA. Higher baseline MSNA, measured by peroneal microneurography, can be found in awake patients with chronic OSA.

Carotid atherosclerosis

An intriguing line of research has identified heavy snoring as an independent factor in carotid, but not femoral, atherosclerosis, with arterial intima-media thickening postulated to result from the mechanical transmission of vibratory pressure waves from upper airway collapse.[4] Of note, these findings have not been extrapolated to a relationship between snoring and carotid artery thromboembolic stroke.

Sleep deprivation

Finally, sleep deprivation is increasingly recognized as an independent factor in morbidity and mortality. Recurrent respiratory events and microarousals may result in overall reduction in total sleep time, sleep fragmentation and sleep architecture changes due to more frequent sleep state transitions, including shifts in total percentages of REM versus NREM sleep, including slow-wave sleep (SWS). The physiological importance of different sleep states is an area of active investigation, but sympathetic activation is characteristic of REM sleep, while SWS may be a "restorative" sleep state. Further studies will undoubtedly help elucidate the causal direction of the complex interrelation between sleep state architecture and the autonomic nervous system.

Clinical presentation

History (Box 6.1)

Excessive daytime sleepiness (EDS)

Perhaps the most common symptom that the SDB patient brings to the attention of their healthcare provider is EDS. It is widely believed that EDS results from sleep fragmentation secondary to recurrent microarousals during sleep. In the case of severe OSA, this is greater than 30 events per hour, or more than once every 2 min throughout the night. As a result, patients wake up unrefreshed and report undesirable sleepiness at inappropriate times including, in severe cases, falling asleep while

---

Box 6.1 Symptoms of sleep-disordered breathing

Nocturnal	Daytime
Reported by patient or witness	Reported by patient
Snoring	Excessive daytime sleepiness*
Witnessed apnea	Morning headache
Gasping/choking	Memory loss
Nocturia	Impaired attention or concentration
Non-restorative sleep	Irritability
Sleep fragmentation/ nighttime awakenings	Loss of libido

*Screening questionnaires: Epworth Sleepiness Scale ($>= 10/24$ is abnormal); STOP-BANG (>3 indicates high risk for OSA); Berlin questionnaire (OSA-specific, high versus low OSA risk stratification in primary care and sleep clinic patients).

---

driving or during conversations. New research points to a possible genetic predisposition towards hypersomnolence in OSA patients, mechanistically distinct from sleep fragmentation. The molecular pathways and pathophysiology of this intriguing hypothesis remain to be elucidated.

☆ TIPS AND TRICKS

History of nocturnal OSA symptoms, including snoring and witnessed apnea, should be obtained from reliable bed partners, as patients are frequently unaware of their symptoms. Similarly, collateral history regarding daytime symptoms may be revealing, as patients often minimize EDS.

The Epworth Sleepiness Scale (ESS) provides a helpful tool for quantifying sleepiness and has been widely adopted as a component of screening questionnaires for OSA, with values greater than 10 out of 24 possible points considered abnormal. Of note, while the ESS may be specific if additional history and physical findings are supportive of OSA, it may not be as sensitive. In other words, while a high ESS score may be consistent with OSA in the appropriate clinical context, a low ESS score should not allay the practitioner's suspicion, as patients may mis- or underperceive their symptoms or misinterpret the questionnaire itself. Regardless of the limitations of the ESS, the questionnaire is commonly required by insurance companies for polysomnography (PSG) and portable monitor testing before authorization.

The Berlin Questionnaire is an OSA-specific questionnaire that has been validated for assigning high versus low risk of OSA to patients in primary care and sleep medicine clinics. The STOP-BANG questionnaire is another screening tool which incorporates self-reported physical signs, including Body Mass Index (BMI) and neck circumference, as predictive factors of OSA risk. This questionnaire was developed for preoperative screening but has not been validated in the clinic setting, even though sensitivity and specificity appear to be higher than those of the ESS.

Snoring

Many OSA patients are not aware of how often or how loudly they snore, or that they snore at all. It is usually the bed partner who, exasperated by the heavy snoring or worried by witnessed cessation of breathing, insists that the patient seek an evaluation for OSA and a remedy for the snoring. It is important to keep in mind that snoring and OSA are considered to be extremes on a spectrum of sleep-disordered breathing, and thus do not always overlap. This is particularly relevant to women, and especially postmenopausal women, in whom the incidence of OSA increases significantly but who may not snore, or may snore softly, and still carry a severe apnea burden.

> ### ✋ CAUTION
>
> While snoring is a common presenting symptom of OSA, snoring may not be present or may be intermittent and soft in postmenopausal women, despite increasing OSA incidence in this population.

Sleep fragmentation, insomnia and other symptoms

If the respiratory event severity is high enough, or the arousal threshold low enough, the OSA patient may awaken themselves gasping for air or choking. These symptoms often lead to an evaluation for gastro-esophageal reflux disease and cardiopulmonary disorders such as asthma or paroxysmal nocturnal dyspnea and orthopnea in decompensated CHF. Often patients report waking up "for no clear reason," and thus may present with complaints of fragmented sleep or sleep maintenance insomnia; the latter is often co-morbid with or secondary to OSA. Nocturia is frequently reported, and while patients often interpret awakening to urinate as a consequence of bladder distension, studies have shown an independent association between nocturia and SDB. Dry mouth and nasal congestion are additional symptoms not typically volunteered, but commonly elicited on direct questioning. Suspicion for OSA is especially appropriate when there is a direct historical correlation between severity of symptoms and weight change, i.e. heavier snoring or worsening EDS in the context of weight gain and vice versa.

Historical red flags in neurological populations (Table 6.1)

Difficulties with attention and concentration, irritability, and working and short-term memory impairment are common complaints in neurological patients. While these may be manifestations of primary neurological disorders or side-effects of medication, OSA should be considered as a potential etiology given an appropriate clinical context.[5] Epilepsy patients present another group of particular interest, as there is some evidence that OSA is associated with late-onset epilepsy as well as increase in seizure frequency that is otherwise unexplained.[6] Sleep deprivation, a well-known risk factor for lowering of the seizure threshold, and increased sleep-wake transitions associated with arousals are two potential mechanisms relating OSA and seizure frequency. Patients with headaches are another population vulnerable to the consequences of OSA. Morning headaches are a common complaint of OSA patients. However, untreated OSA is also known to exacerbate primary headaches, including complex and common migraine, and cluster headache.

Populations at high risk for sleep-disordered breathing (Box 6.2)

These include obese patients, especially those with a large neck size, and formal preoperative evaluation for OSA is recommended by the American Academy of Sleep Medicine (AASM) prior to bariatric surgery.

Table 6.1 Symptoms and characteristics of primary neurological disorders which should prompt consideration for sleep-disordered breathing screening

Neurological diagnosis	Characteristics or neurological symptoms
Ischemic stroke* or transient ischemic attack*	Refractory hypertension* (requiring =>3 agents) Arrhythmias* (atrial fibrillation, ventricular) CHF or reduced left ventricular ejection fraction* Diabetes mellitus II* Internal carotid artery stenosis and heavy snoring
Epilepsy	Nocturnal Late onset Refractory* or unexplained increase in frequency
Primary headache	Chronic daily headache, especially morning* Cluster*and hypnic headache Unexplained exacerbation of long-standing migraine*, tension*, posttraumatic* headaches
Neuromuscular disorders	Early onset (i.e. Duchenne muscular dystrophy)
Demyelinating disease	Multiple sclerosis (involvement of brainstem respiratory drive centers)
Neurodegenerative disorders	Alzheimer's disease* (pre- or early symptomatic) Vascular dementia Multiple system atrophy and stridor

*Evidence suggests that OSA treatment may improve outcomes in these disorders.

Box 6.2 Risk factors for sleep-disordered breathing

Anatomy
BMI >35 kg/m^2
Neck circumference:
  >17 inches men
  >16 inches women
Craniofacial anatomical variants:
  Retrognathia
  Midfacial hypoplasia (e.g. Down's syndrome)
  Tonsillar hypertrophy
  Crowded posterior oropharynx

Demographics
Age >50
Men or postmenopausal women
Asian or African American
Family history of sleep-disordered breathing

Medical conditions
Congestive heart failure
Pulmonary hypertension
Type 2 diabetes (obesity, diabetic neuropathy)

Neurological conditions
Stroke or transient ischemic attack
Neuromuscular disorders (including, but not limited to):
  Motor neuron disorders
  Neuropathy (including diabetic neuropathy, chronic inflammatory demyelinating polyradiculoneuropathy)
  Myasthenia gravis
  Myopathy (myotonic dystrophy type I, Duchenne muscular dystrophy)
Epilepsy
Neurodegenerative disorders
  Alzheimer's disease
  Vascular dementia
  Multiple system atrophy
Brainstem insults (stroke, tumor, demyelination, infection)

Other high-risk groups include patients with craniofacial anatomy resulting in a narrow airway, including but not limited to retrognathia, micrognathia, mandibular, and midfacial hypoplasia as seen in Down's and Marfan's syndromes; older patients, as the prevalence of OSA increases with age and is estimated to triple in individuals older than 65; men, who are affected by OSA three times more frequently than women; postmenopausal women, who develop the same incidence of OSA as men, suggesting protective effects of reproductive hormones; Asian and African American populations, who are at higher risk of developing OSA even in the absence of obesity or increased neck width; and patients with family history of SDB, as OSA appears to have heritable components. Finally, populations at high risk of morbidity or mortality from untreated OSA, including commercial truck drivers and public transportation drivers, merit screening for SDB.

> **✋ CAUTION**
>
> Obstructive sleep apea is defined as AHI >5 events/hour in the presence of symptoms, or AHI >15 events/hour in asymptomatic patients. It is important to maintain a high level of clinical suspicion in populations at high risk for OSA, as treatment is indicated in asymptomatic patients for prevention of co-morbid cardio- and cerebrovascular disease.

> **★ TIPS AND TRICKS**
>
> Unexplained exacerbations of primary neurological conditions may be secondary to co-morbid SDB and respond to CPAP treatment. Symptoms may include worsening primary headache (cluster, hypnic, migraine, tension, chronic daily, and posttraumatic headache), refractory epilepsy or increasing seizure frequency, and impaired memory and attention.

Neurological populations with high prevalence of SDB include patients with motor neuron disorders; neuromuscular junction pathology, such as myasthenia gravis; neuropathy, especially diabetic neuropathy; congenital and acquired myopathies, including muscular dystrophies, especially myotonic dystrophy type 1 and Duchenne muscular dystrophy (DMD); epilepsy [7]; and neurodegenerative disorders, including Alzheimer's disease (AD), vascular dementia, and multiple system atrophy (MSA). Of note, many neurological disorders, certainly ones involving the brainstem respiratory centers, such as multiple sclerosis, may result in CSA, characterized by cessation of airflow and lack of compensatory respiratory drive, instead of or in addition to OSA.[8]

Physical examination

General examination

Vital signs measurement, including height and weight for BMI calculation, neck circumference, blood pressure and pulse oximetry are essential aspects of the physical exam in the patient being evaluated for OSA. BMI >30–35 kg/m² and neck circumference >17 inches (43 cm) in men and >16 inches (40.6 cm) in women are indicators of OSA risk. Hypertension, especially resistant to multiple antihypertensive agents, should raise suspicion for untreated OSA in the absence of alternative etiologies. Hypoxia during the awake state suggests primary pulmonary or cardiovascular processes, with rare exceptions such as severe CCHS, and the likelihood that the patient will require more than just conventional positive airway pressure (PAP) treatment should they be diagnosed with OSA.

Airway examination

A Mallampati or modified Mallampati score of the oropharynx should be obtained by asking the patient to open their mouth as wide as possible and protrude their tongue, versus keep the tongue in the oral cavity for the Modified Mallampati. A score of 3 or 4 is a risk factor for both presence and severity of OSA. The oropharynx should be evaluated for any structural elements leading to narrowing of the airway, including anatomical variants, such as lateral pharyngeal wall or peritonsillar narrowing, tonsillar or adenoid hypertrophy, a low-lying elongated soft palate, a long, edematous uvula, macroglossia with or without scalloping or notching of the tongue, retro- or micrognathia, overjet, congenital craniofacial malformations (for example, midface hypoplasia as seen in Down's patients), or evidence of anatomical remodeling by long-standing OSA, including a high-arched, narrow hard palate or maxillary restriction. The nasal passages should be inspected for nasal septal deviation, nasal polyps, turbinate hypertrophy, or mucosal erythema consistent with rhinitis.

Diagnosis

Diagnostic approach

Objective testing for OSA is indicated in symptomatic patients, i.e. those reporting EDS or cognitive dysfunction, with history and physical findings placing them at high risk of OSA. However, given the potential cardiovascular, cerebrovascular and metabolic consequences of moderate-to-severe OSA, objective testing should be performed even in the non-sleepy patient who is at risk for and/or reports nocturnal symptoms of OSA, including snoring, sleep fragmentation, and nocturnal dyspnea. Objective testing is indicated to establish the severity of OSA, as this will dictate therapeutic choices, and treatment is recommended in asymptomatic patients with moderate-to-severe OSA.

⚠ CAUTION

Portable monitor (PM) studies may underestimate the severity of apnea because cortical arousals cannot be evaluated given the lack of EEG recording, and the lack of accurate total sleep time (TST) measurement may overestimate TST and underpower the number of respiratory events per hour of sleep time. Therefore, if clinical suspicion or pretest probability for OSA is high, a PSG is indicated if an initial PM study does not meet diagnostic criteria for OSA.

The following high-risk patients should undergo objective testing for OSA in the presence of nocturnal or daytime symptoms: obese patients; patients with history of stroke or transient ischemic attack; patients with diastolic or systolic heart failure, particularly if nocturnal symptoms are present despite optimal medical management; patients with coronary artery disease or cardiac arrhythmias, especially atrial fibrillation or ventricular arrhythmias; patients with medically refractory hypertension. Sleep studies are also routinely indicated as part of the preoperative evaluation prior to upper airway surgery for snoring or OSA, as well as prior to bariatric surgery. Follow-up sleep studies are indicated to assess treatment response to non-PAP modalities, including airway surgery for moderate-to-severe OSA, oral appliances (OA), expiratory resistance nasal valves, or if OSA symptoms recur while on treatment, despite initial response. Follow-up sleep studies are also indicated for patients on PAP therapy after significant (10% of body weight or more) weight loss or weight gain with return of symptoms, insufficient clinical improvement, or recurrence of OSA symptoms despite initial resolution with PAP therapy. There is no indication for a repeat sleep study in patients with persistent resolution of symptoms on continued PAP therapy.

In-laboratory PSG and home testing with PMs are the two methods available for objective testing of OSA. PSG is indicated for all types of SDB. PM testing can be used for OSA diagnosis when there is a high pretest probability for moderate-to-severe OSA after a comprehensive sleep evaluation by a sleep specialist. However, PM studies may underestimate the severity of apnea given the lack of EEG recording and thus the inability to evaluate for cortical arousals, which are incorporated in hypopnea scoring in PSGs. PMs also lack accurate TST measurements and allow for overestimation of TST, thus potentially underpowering the AHI, defined as the number of respiratory events per hour of sleep time. Therefore, if clinical suspicion or pretest probability for OSA is high, a PSG is indicated if an initial PM study does not meet diagnostic criteria for OSA.

Unattended PM studies may be inaccurate and therefore not appropriate for diagnosis of OSA in patients with neuromuscular disorders, CHF, especially class III or IV, and pulmonary disease. PMs may be used for OSA diagnosis in patients who cannot tolerate in-laboratory PSG secondary to immobility, safety issues, or critical illness. PSG is the indicated form of objective testing and diagnosis in patients with suspected CSA, or other primary sleep disorders, including narcolepsy or other hypersomnias, periodic limb movement disorder (PLMD) or parasomnias.

Sleep study modalities

Polysomnography

The following physiological measurements are required for the PSG diagnosis of OSA: EEG channels, electrooculogram (EOG), EMG, and recordings of airflow, oxygen saturation, respiratory effort, and heart rate, or an electrocardiogram (ECG). A limited EEG montage is typically used, often with two central, two frontal and two occipital channels and ear references. A full 10–20 EEG montage can be used if seizure is suspected, but is not part of the standard PSG. Two EOG channels record both vertical and horizontal eye movements. EMG of the chin or mentalis muscle is used to stage sleep, assessing for atonia during REM sleep. Additional anterior tibialis EMG recording is recommended and typically used to assess for movement arousals and periodic limb movements of sleep. A couple of methods for measuring airflow are used: an oronasal thermal sensor detects changes in air temperature with inhalation or exhalation, and is sensitive for complete apneas but may miss hypopneas; a nasal pressure transducer is more sensitive for detecting decreased airflow with hypopneas and can indicate increased upper airway resistance by a squaring of the otherwise rounded flow signal. Respiratory effort is measured by chest and abdominal belts using piezo crystal-based or inductance plethysmography technology. Finally, body position and snoring are typically tracked. Esophageal manometry and end-tidal CO_2 are available, but not routinely used in adult PSG.

A full night diagnostic PSG can be used for SDB diagnosis, followed by a dedicated titration study on a separate night where the optimal PAP modality and pressure are determined. However, if an AHI >20–40 is documented during the first 2 hours of a diagnostic study, a split-night study may be performed instead, where PAP is titrated on the same night.

Portable monitor testing

There are a variety of PMs but we will focus on type 3 devices, which allow for portable testing for sleep apnea. Type 3 PMs typically monitor a minimum of four physiological parameters, including airflow, respiratory effort, oxygen saturation, and heart rate. The same technologies used in PSGs should be employed in PM testing, i.e. oronasal thermistor and nasal pressure transducer for airflow measurement, inductance plethysmography chest and abdomen belts for respiratory effort, pulse oximetry for oxygen saturation, and ECG for heart rate measurements. PM testing does not include EEG, EOG or EMG, and body position is sometimes, but not always, monitored. Because EEG is not recorded, arousal hypopneas cannot be scored, and respiratory events have to be normalized to study time, instead of sleep time, to derive the AHI. These factors lower the sensitivity of PM studies for SDB detection and accurate estimate of SDB severity.

Diagnostic criteria

Obstructive sleep apnea severity is quantified using the Apnea Hypopnea Index (AHI) or Respiratory Disturbance Index (RDI). Apneas and hypopneas are defined as >90% and >30% reduction in airflow amplitude respectively, lasting a minimum of 10 sec, in association with oxygen desaturation of at least 4% (Medicare criteria), or 3% and/or an EEG arousal (AASM criteria). The AHI represents the number of respiratory events per hour of sleep time. In addition to apneas and hypopneas, the RDI incorporates

RERAs, again normalized to hours of sleep. A diagnosis of OSA can be made in patients with any daytime (i.e. sleepiness) or nocturnal (witnessed snoring or apneas, nocturnal arousals) symptoms and an AHI or RDI >5. An AHI or RDI >15 bestows the diagnosis of OSA even in the absence of symptoms.

Thus, an AHI or RDI of 0–4.9 is considered to be within normal limits, 5–14 is indicative of mild, 15–30 moderate, and above 30 severe apnea. As mentioned previously, since PMs do not incorporate EEG recording, cortical arousals cannot be used as a scoring criterion, and the duration of sleep time may be overestimated, consequently underestimating the AHI and lowering the sensitivity of PM testing. Of note, body position tracking in both PSG and PM testing should be used to assess for positional apnea and thus inform treatment choices. Sleep staging in PSG recording can be used to assess for REM versus NREM-predominant SDB, as NREM-predominant SDB may raise suspicion for CSA.

In addition to sleep staging and TST, the PSG EEG tracing allows for quantification of sleep onset latency (SOL), wake after sleep onset (WASO) time, REM onset latency (ROL), and sleep efficiency calculation, providing some indication of sleep quality within the constraints of the first-night effect, or possible sleep alteration by an unfamiliar environment.

Management of obstructive sleep apnea

Obstructive sleep apnea is a chronic disease, requiring long-term management best achieved by specialized multidisciplinary healthcare teams.[9] Multiple treatments have been developed including positive airway pressure, oral appliances, and surgery.

> ★ **TIPS AND TRICKS**
>
> Expected improvement in sleep quality and EDS secondary to OSA treatment should be emphasized, as it may improve initial patient compliance with therapy.

Positive airway pressure

This is the gold standard therapy for mild, moderate, and severe OSA. It only became available as recently as 1981, but can now be delivered by a multitude of modalities, including continuous (CPAP), bi-level (BPAP), and auto-titrating (APAP) modes. Compliance metrics during the first 4–8 weeks of PAP therapy, in particular, are predictive of future compliance, and quick and effective trouble-shooting for any problems encountered by the patient is crucial.

Continuous positive airway pressure

Continuous positive airway pressure is indicated as first-line therapy in OSA as well as treatment-emergent sleep apnea and CSR-CSA. The optimal pressure in centimeters of water can be determined during a split-night study in many cases. When significant co-morbidities are present, including CHF, primary CSA or pulmonary disease, a dedicated titration study is recommended. A repeat titration study is indicated in patients with treatment-emergent complex apnea to monitor response to therapy at 4–6 weeks after initiation of CPAP. Although larger studies have not found that BPAP or APAP modes are better tolerated than CPAP on average, it is possible that individual patients, whom we cannot currently identify prior to exposure to PAP, can tolerate BPAP or APAP better than the fixed pressure of CPAP.

Bi-level positive airway pressure

Bi-level positive airway pressure delivers different pressures during inspiration, when pressure requirements are higher, and expiration. BPAP provides an optional therapy in CPAP-intolerant patients and should be considered especially when high pressure is needed, which may be difficult to exhale against. Pressure reduction during expiration (pressure relief) can be added to the above PAP modes as needed in order to improve compliance.

Auto-titrating positive airway pressure

Auto-titrating positive airway pressure detect changes in airflow due to obstruction and increase or decrease pressure as needed over the course of the night. It can be initiated in patients without major medical co-morbidities, including uncontrolled hypertension, CHF, CSA or pulmonary disease, who have been diagnosed with OSA by PM testing, and have not had a titration study. APAP may also be indicated in situations of anticipated change in weight or other physiological parameters, such as pregnancy, patients with recurrent myasthenia gravis exacerbations, patients with large pressure requirement changes that are positional in nature, or following bariatric or upper airway surgery.

Adaptive servo-ventilation

Adaptive servo-ventilation (ASV) is indicated in patients with OSA and CSA, including treatment-emergent sleep apnea, who have failed CPAP. The ASV mode aims to improve ventilatory stability and minimize periodic breathing. It does so by automatically adjusting the pressure to 90% of the most recent average minute ventilation requirement, which is continuously monitored.

General points on positive airway pressure

Factors which commonly contribute to PAP intolerance include oronasal dryness or irritation, which can be alleviated by the humidification chambers incorporated in most new PAP machines; nasal congestion or rhinitis, treatable with nasal steroid sprays, humidification and decongestants; difficulties with mask habituation leading to sleep initiation and/or maintenance insomnia. The most appropriate facial interface, ranging from nasal cushions to a full oronasal mask, can help alleviate habituation difficulties. In cases of significant insomnia, a trial of hypnotic medication may be indicated, not only for sleep initiation insomnia but for sleep stabilization, as both will help with PAP habituation. Of note, any hypnotics with muscle relaxation properties, such as benzodiazepines, are contraindicated in OSA patients not using PAP, as they may worsen apnea severity.

Behavioral interventions

Modifiable risk factors for airway collapse can reduce the severity of SDB to various degrees depending on the underlying OSA pathophysiology.

Weight loss

Weight loss is likely to reduce OSA severity in overweight or obese patients. Dietary approaches as well as evaluation for bariatric surgery in the morbidly obese are both encouraged. However, given the low success rate of behavioral weight reduction and the incomplete cure rate of OSA by weight loss alone, PAP treatment should be initiated concurrently, with follow-up PSG or titration study performed after weight loss of 10% or more of body weight.

Positional therapy

Positional therapy, typically with avoidance of the supine position, may be particularly helpful in cases of objectively proven positional apnea by PSG or PM testing. Various commercially available or home-made products may be used, including wedge pillows, tennis balls or pressure-activated alarms sewn on the back of a nightshirt. Objective position monitoring and resolution of symptoms should be instituted if this is chosen as the only form of OSA therapy.

Avoidance of muscle relaxants

Avoidance of muscle relaxants, including late-night alcohol ingestion or benzodiazepine use at bedtime, is recommended. One exception is the use of hypnotics by the sleep specialist in order to consolidate and stabilize sleep for improvement of PAP compliance.

Oral appliances

Oral appliances (OA) aim to reduce airway collapsibility by advancing the mandible or the tongue with respect to the resting state. Mandibular repositioning appliances (MRA) cover both upper and lower teeth and advance the mandible, while tongue retaining devices (TRD) advance the tongue only. These devices need to be custom fitted and typically require multiple visits to the dentist for gradual adjustment. OAs are only indicated for treatment of moderate-to-severe OSA for patients who have failed PAP or other OSA therapies. However, OAs are less efficacious than PAP, achieving success in approximately 50% of OSA patients. Therefore, a follow-up sleep study is indicated once OA therapy has been optimized to objectively evaluate effectiveness.

Nasal expiratory positive airway pressure

This is a relatively new FDA-approved modality for the treatment of OSA. Expiratory resistance nasal valves attach externally to each nostril and act as one-way resistors, allowing free airflow during inspiration but increasing expiratory nasal resistance by restricting airflow to small openings only. The result is expiratory PAP only, as opposed to the continual pressure provided during PAP therapy. As clinical response cannot be predicted, a follow-up sleep study is indicated for objective evaluation of therapy effectiveness.

Medication

Medication can be used in conjunction with PAP. REM-suppressing agents, including tricyclic antidepressants and selective serotonin reuptake inhibitors, may improve OSA severity by reducing the fraction of REM sleep when OSA is typically exacerbated by atonia, but the effect is small. Modafinil is indicated in OSA patients who have persistent EDS despite optimal OSA PAP treatment, and in whom no alternative cause of sleepiness can be identified.

> **⚠ CAUTION**
>
> Benzodiazepines are contraindicated in untreated OSA because of their muscle relaxant properties, but can be used to facilitate CPAP habituation in patients with anxiety or insomnia.

Surgical interventions

Multiple surgeries have been developed to try to target and open the site of airway collapse. Surgeries for OSA, including but not limited to nasal (septoplasty, polypectomy, turbinate reduction), oropharyngeal (tonsillectomy and/or adenoidectomy, uvulopalatopharyngoplasty [UPPP]), maxillomandibular advancement (MMA) and hypopharyngeal (tongue reduction or advancement) procedures, should be considered in medically refractory patients. Discussion of the details of the individual surgeries is beyond the scope of this chapter. In general, airway surgery for OSA has an approximate success rate of 50–60% in adults, with the exception of MMA, which results in definitive OSA cure in 95% of cases.

Emerging therapies

Clinical trials are currently under way testing hypoglossal nerve stimulation and continuous oral negative pressure as alternative OSA therapies.

Outcome variables

Once medical therapy is initiated, patients should be continually evaluated for resolution of nocturnal (snoring, sleep fragmentation) and daytime (sleepiness) symptoms; quality of life measures such as increased energy, improved concentration, and patient and spousal satisfaction; therapy compliance; appropriate sleep hygiene and adequate sleep; and improvement in medical co-morbidities, such as refractory hypertension.

Management of central sleep apnea

The central tenet of treating CSA in CHF is to maximize heart failure therapy and cardiac function. Improving cardiac function reduces CSA. However, CSA may also contribute to deterioration of cardiac function and should be treated if CSA persists despite maximal therapy. Typically, treatment-emergent CSA will resolve over time as the patient adapts to PAP therapy. If not, specific therapy may be tried to resolve the CSA.[10]

Positive airway pressure therapy

Continuous positive airway pressure

Continuous positive airway pressure is indicated for the initial treatment of CSA related to CHF and has been shown to improve transplant-free survival in patients whose AHI is normalized by CPAP. If the CPAP level is set empirically, rather than by titration, a repeat sleep study is needed to demonstrate effectiveness and CPAP should be stopped if CSA is not eliminated as this group may actually have reduced survival. CPAP may also be effective for other types of CSA but, again, effectiveness must be demonstrated.

Bi-level positive airway pressure

In the spontaneous timed mode, a setting that delivers a fixed number of breaths if the patient does not breathe on their own, BPAP may be effective for CSA related to CHF. Given its lower rate of effectiveness, this mode of PAP should only be used after trials with CPAP and ASV have been unsuccessful.

Auto-titrating positive airway pressure

Auto-titrating positive airway pressure is currently not indicated for treatment of CSA.

Adaptive servo-ventilation

Adaptive servo-ventilation has been shown to improve the AHI and left ventricular ejection fraction (LVEF) in CHF patients with CSA. Outcome data for ASV are comparable to CPAP in these patients but the cost of the device is considerably higher. ASV has also been used in treatment-emergent CSA.

Oxygen therapy

Although the mechanism of action is unclear, supplemental oxygen can be effective in treating CSA in CHF patients. Oxygen has beneficial effects in reducing AHI and improving LVEF and is better tolerated than CPAP.

Medication

Additional agents specifically used for CSA treatment include acetazolamide, which appears to decrease ventilator instability in CSA, presumably by modifying the apnea threshold through induced hypercarbia. Ironically, barbiturates may be helpful in CSA despite their effect as respiratory suppressants, as they appear to result in increased genioglossus activity and may consolidate sleep, thus reducing sleep-wake transitions when CSA is most likely to occur. Zolpidem and triazolam may be considered for the treatment of primary CSA to try to increase the arousal threshold and reduce sleep fragmentation. These agents should be used only in those patients without risk factors for respiratory depression.

Outcomes in neurological patients with sleep-disordered breathing

Patients who are likely to benefit from treatment of previously unrecognized OSA, and also of particular relevance to the neurologist, include those with a history of prior stroke or transient ischemic attack (TIA), as compliance with CPAP OSA treatment results in reduced mortality in ischemic stroke and TIA patients[11]; treatment-refractory hypertension, where a dose-dependent reduction in systolic and diastolic blood pressures with longer hours of nightly CPAP use has been demonstrated in a small group of patients[12]; CHF, atrial fibrillation, and poorly controlled diabetes. There is emerging evidence that OSA patients compliant with CPAP therapy experience improvement in cluster,[13] migraine, tension, and chronic posttraumatic headaches.[14] Limited data suggest that CPAP may slow cognitive decline in Alzheimer's disease patients with OSA,[15] as well as reducing seizure frequency in patients with epilepsy and co-morbid OSA.

Conclusion

The importance of having a high index of suspicion, screening for, and treating SDB in patients at risk is increasingly recognized. Untreated SDB is associated with increased morbidity and mortality in patients with ischemic stroke and cardiovascular disease. The link appears to be causal, as it persists when confounders are accounted for, and the health consequences are proportional to the severity of SDB. SDB negatively impacts preexisting hypertension, cardiac arrhythmias including atrial fibrillation and ventricular arrhythmias, and insulin resistance. Neurologists need to be aware of patients with primary neurological disorders at high risk of co-morbid SDB, including those with ischemic stroke or TIA, refractory or nocturnal epilepsy, demyelinating disorders (multiple sclerosis), headache (common and complex migraine, chronic daily, morning, cluster, hypnic, tension and chronic posttraumatic headaches), neuromuscular disorders (motor neuron disorders, neuropathy, myasthenia gravis, myopathy, especially myotonic dystrophy type I and DMD), and neurodegenerative disease (Alzheimer's dementia, vascular demenia, and MSA).

References

1. St Louis EK. Diagnosing and treating co-morbid sleep apnea in neurological disorders. *Pract Neurol* 2010; **9**: 26–30.

2. Marin JM, Carrizo SJ, Vicente E, Agusti AG. Long-term cardiovascular outcomes in men with obstructive sleep apnoea-hypopnoea with or without treatment with continuous positive airway pressure: an observational study. *Lancet* 2005; **365**: 1046–53.

3. Young T, Finn L, Peppard PE, et al. Sleep disordered breathing and mortality: eighteen-year follow-up of the Wisconsin sleep cohort. *Sleep* 2008; **31**: 1071–8.

4. Lee SA, Amis TC, Byth K, et al. Heavy snoring as a cause of carotid artery atherosclerosis. *Sleep* 2008; **31**: 1207–13.

5. Ho ML, Brass SD. Obstructive sleep apnea. *Neurol Int* 2011; **3**: e15.

6. Chihorek AM, Abou-Khalil B, Malow BA. Obstructive sleep apnea is associated with seizure occurrence in older adults with epilepsy. *Neurology* 2007; **69**: 1823–7.

7. Foldvary-Schaefer N, Andrews ND, Pornsriniyom D, Moul DE, Sun Z, Bena J. Sleep apnea and epilepsy: who's at risk? *Epilepsy Behav* 2012; **25**: 363–7.

8. Braley TJ, Segal BM, Chervin RD. Sleep-disordered breathing in multiple sclerosis. *Neurology* 2012; **79**: 929–36.

9. Epstein LJ, Kristo D, Strollo PJ Jr, et al. Clinical guideline for the evaluation, management and long-term care of obstructive sleep apnea in adults. *J Clin Sleep Med* 2009; **5**: 263–76.

10. Aurora RN, Chowdhuri S, Ramar K, et al.The treatment of central sleep apnea syndromes in adults: practice parameters with an evidence-based literature review and meta-analyses. *Sleep* 2012; **35**: 17–40.

11. Martinez-Garcia MA, Soler-Cataluna JJ, Ejarque-Martinez L, et al. Continuous positive airway pressure treatment reduces mortality in patients with ischemic stroke and obstructive sleep apnea: a 5-year follow-up study. *Am J Respir Crit Care Med* 2009; **180**: 36–41.

12. Lozano L, Tovar JL, Sampol G, et al. Continuous positive airway pressure treatment in sleep apnea patients with resistant hypertension: a randomized, controlled trial. *J Hypertension* 2010; **28**: 2161–8.

13. Nath Zallek S, Chervin RD. Improvement in cluster headache after treatment for obstructive sleep apnea. *Sleep Med* 2000; **1**: 135–8.

14. Johnson KG, Ziemba AM, Garb JL. Improvement in headaches with continuous positive airway pressure for obstructive sleep apnea: a retrospective analysis. *Headache* 2013; **53**: 333–43.

15. Cooke JR, Ayalon L, Palmer BW, et al. Sustained use of CPAP slows deterioration of cognition, sleep, and mood in patients with Alzheimer's disease and obstructive sleep apnea: a preliminary study. *J Clin Sleep Med* 2009; **5**: 305–9.

7

Surgical Management of Sleep-Disordered Breathing

Masayoshi Takashima, MD, FACS, FAAOA,[1] Jaime Gateno, DDS, MD,[2,3] Melinda Davis-Malessevich, MD,[1] and Robert Busch, DMD, MD[2]

[1]The Bobby R Alford Department of Otolaryngology – Head and Neck Surgery, Baylor College of Medicine, USA
[2]Weill Cornell Medical College, USA
[3]Oral and Maxillofacial Surgery Department, The Methodist Hospital Physician Organization, USA

Surgical evaluation

The purpose of this evaluation is to gather all the necessary information to determine appropriate surgical treatment for patients with snoring, upper airway resistance syndrome or obstructive sleep apnea. It consists of three parts: a pertinent medical history, a focused physical examination, and the evaluation of ancillary studies, which includes either a home or laboratory polysomnography. During this process, careful attention should be paid to the presence of co-morbidities and the severity of the obstructive sleep apnea, as well as assessing to what degree the patient is symptomatic from this disorder.

Pertinent history

Excessive daytime sleepiness (EDS) is a common complaint in Western society, and is estimated to be present in up to 40% of the total population.[1,2] Excessive sleepiness may result from both physiological causes, such as sleep deprivation related to irregular sleep-wake schedule, and pathological causes, such as obstructive sleep apnea (OSA). The spectrum of sleep-disordered breathing ranges from upper airway resistance syndrome to frank obstruction. OSA is characterized by episodes of partial or complete upper airway collapse leading to cessation or reduction of airflow.[3,4] Such events lead to oxygen desaturation and sleep fragmentation, causing excessive daytime sleepiness, morning headaches, depression, memory loss, impaired alertness, decreased libido, and reduced cognitive function.

A thorough history is the first step in evaluating a patient with complaints of EDS (Box 7.1). The bed partner, caregiver or parents of children are often the most helpful historians. The patient and family should be queried about snoring, restless sleep, choking or gasping episodes, and awakenings during sleep. Nocturnal perspiration, nocturia, teeth grinding, and symptoms of nocturnal gastroesophageal reflux are also commonly associated with OSA. Other pertinent parts of the history include asking about paresthesias, uncontrollable limb movements at sleep onset, hypnogogic hallucinations, cataplexy, irregular sleep-wake cycle, delayed sleep onset, and family history of sleep disorders, all of which may suggest another cause for the patient's EDS.[4,5]

The Epworth Sleepiness Scale (ESS) is a simple, self-administered questionnaire that provides a general subjective measure of daytime sleepiness, which has been validated in patients with OSA. The patient is asked to score on a scale of 0–3 the likelihood of falling asleep in eight situations, with 0 being no chance of dozing off and 3 being a high chance of dozing off. The scores for the eight

Sleep Medicine in Neurology, First Edition. Edited by Douglas B. Kirsch.
© 2014 John Wiley & Sons, Ltd. Published 2014 by John Wiley & Sons, Ltd.

Box 7.1 Elevated risk factors
for obstructive sleep apnea

- Age greater than 65 years
- Neck circumference greater than 17 inches in men and 16 inches in women
- Body Mass Index (BMI) greater than 30 kg/m²
- Hypertension, cardiovascular disease
- Male gender
- Postmenopausal female
- African American or Asian race[3,6,7]

Box 7.2 Anatomical areas of interest

- High-arched hard palate
- Tongue crenations/large tongue
- Low-hanging soft palate (unable to see the tonsillar arches)
- Loss of hyoid-mental angle
- Micrognathia/retrognathia
- Craniofacial abnormalities
- Narrow tonsillar pillars/tonsillar enlargement

questions are added together to obtain a single number. A number in the 0–9 range is considered to be normal, and anything 10 or above is suggestive of sleep-disordered breathing. Although suggestive, the ESS is not a diagnostic tool in isolation, and is thus used primarily as a screening tool. In a group of approximately 1800 subjects, the mean score in those without OSA was 7.2 and in those with OSA was 9.3.[5,8] Furthermore, treating OSA with continuous positive airway pressure has been shown to improve ESS scores by a mean of 3.8 points.[9]

Focused physical examination

The focused physical examination of a patient with suspected or diagnosed OSA usually starts with an inspection of the head and neck (Box 7.2). An intranasal exam is initially performed to evaluate the adequacy of the nasal passage. Nasal congestion from allergic causes should be addressed medically.

✩ TIPS AND TRICKS

Medical management of nasal congestion

- Nasal saline irrigations
- Nasal steroids
- Nasal antihistamines
- Cromolyn nasal spray
- Oral antihistamines
- Anti-leukotrienes
- Temporary measures:
  - Oral decongestants
  - Nasal decongestant sprays

Enlarged inferior turbinates, a nasoseptal deviation, nasal valve collapse or nasal obstruction from nasal polyps should be documented. Unobstructed nasal breathing is an important initial component for obtaining surgical cure of OSA and thus is usually addressed first. Another benefit of proceeding with nasal surgery first is that by decreasing upper airway/nasal resistance, frequently, positive pressure requirements can be lowered, improving mask air leakage and improving continuous positive airway pressure (CPAP) usage compliance. Overall, improvements in nasal breathing have been shown to improve overall quality of life. Patients requiring orthognathic surgery for OSA may also benefit from primary nasal surgery as some procedures may temporarily restrict oral respirations. Once recovered from nasal surgery, CPAP pressures can be retitrated with the intention of lowering pressures and thus improving CPAP compliance. At the time of nasal surgery, a diagnostic, video-recorded sleep endoscopy can be performed to diagnose the anatomical region causing the OSA. These data would be used for surgical planning purposes if further oropharyngeal surgery becomes necessary for the surgical cure of the patient's OSA.

Because the evaluation of the upper airway is subjective, it is difficult to maintain consistent language between examiners. A helpful tool for objectively assessing the oral airway for the presence of obstruction is the Friedman tongue position (FTP) (Figure 7.1a) and tonsil grade (Figure 7.1b).[10] Both grade the anatomical relationship of the tongue with the tonsils, uvula, soft palate, and hard palate. The patient is asked to open the mouth widely without phonating while keeping the tongue in neutral position. This represents the anatomical location of

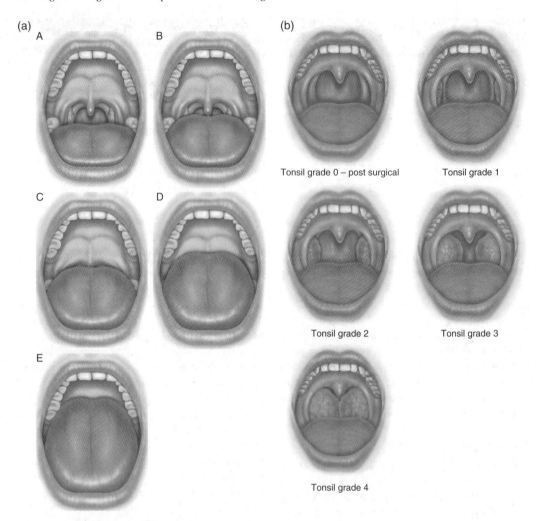

Figure 7.1 (a) Friedman tongue position (FTP). A. FTP I: visualization of the entire uvula and tonsils/pillars. B. FTP IIa: visualization of most of the uvula, but tonsils/pillars are absent. C. FTB IIb: visualization of the entire soft palate to the base of the uvula. D. FTP III: visualization of some of the soft palate, but structures distal to this are not seen. E. FTP IV: visualization of the hard palate only. (b) Tonsil grading system. Reprinted with permission from Dr Michael Friedman.

the tongue and tonsils within the mouth, and is contrasted to the Mallampati classification (an indicator of ease of endotracheal intubation), which requires the patient to protrude the tongue. The reproducibility and accuracy of FTP and tonsil grade were shown to be very good (kappa value 0.82) with consistent strength agreement among residents, fellows, and attendings.[10] When assessing the tongue, inspection of tongue crenations (scalloping of the lateral edges of the tongue from indentations made by the teeth) helps identify the size of the tongue in relation to the space that the tongue occupies. For example, a patient may have a normal-sized tongue but due to a small oral cavity, the tongue may actually be too large, causing an obstruction.

The next area to focus on is the uvula, tonsillar pillars, and the height of the arch of the hard palate. A long, beefy uvula is frequently the cause of loud snoring. Tonsils may be of normal size, but the distance between the tonsillar pillars on each side may impinge on the airway. This finding is frequently due to a high-arched hard palate. Patients with a high

Figure 7.2 Horizontal and vertical occlusal relationships. Molar relationship (A), canine relationship (B), incisal relationship (C), overjet and overbite (*box*).

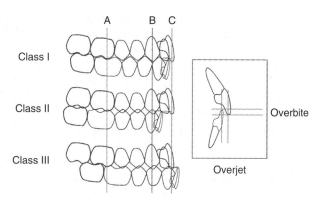

arch tend to have anatomical features of a long anterior-posterior (A-P) oropharyngeal distance but narrow lateral distances. This abnormality typically occurs during the developmental phases of craniofacial skeletal maturation where the high-arched palate does not flatten by widening the distance between opposite molars. Commonly, it is observed in patients with "adenoid facies" where allergies cause nasal congestion, which results in a patient who is a perpetual mouth breather. In a mouth breather, the tongue does not place any pressure onto the hard palate to widen. These patients may benefit from an oral maxillofacial surgical evaluation to assess the need to widen the palate.

Evaluation of the significance of the retrolingual region is quite difficult to ascertain in the awake patient, as the anatomy and tone in an awake patient are very different from those seen in an asleep patient. As awake patients seldom obstruct the airway, examination while the patient is awake may give hints as to the underlying problem but further studies, such as diagnostic sleep endoscopy, are required to accurately pinpoint the exact site of anatomical obstruction. If the retrolingual region is to be assessed with the patient awake, it must be done with the tongue in a neutral position inside the mouth (i.e. patients rarely sleep with the tongue hanging out of the mouth).

The exam should include an evaluation of the facial profile. Clinically, a profile can be classified as straight, convex or concave. A straight facial profile is considered normal. A convex profile is usually associated with mandibular deficiency and in severe cases with decreased retroglossal airway space. A concave profile is usually associated with mandibular excess although it can also be a sign of midface deficiency, a condition that

when severe can be associated with decreased retropalatal airway space.

An important part of the examination of the oral cavity is evaluation of the dental occlusion. The term *dental occlusion* denotes the relationship between the upper and lower teeth when they are in contact. This relationship is usually described in three dimensions: anteroposterior, vertical, and transverse. To assess the occlusion in the anteroposterior dimension, we evaluate three different areas: incisal, canine, and molar. In the incisal area, the anteroposterior relationship of the upper and lower incisors is assessed by measuring the *overjet*, which is the horizontal distance between the edges of the upper and lower central incisors (Figure 7.2). The mean normal overjet is 2 mm. In the canine area, a normal relationship occurs when the embrasure located between the lower canine and first premolar is aligned with the tip of the upper canine (see Figure 7.2). Finally, in the molar area, a normal anteroposterior relationship occurs when the central groove of the lower first molar is aligned with the mesiobuccal cusp of the upper first molar (see Figure 7.2). Any deviation from this normal arrangement produces a malocclusion.

Malocclusions characterized by an abnormal anteroposterior relationship are assessed using the system developed by Angle. In this system, the upper teeth are considered fixed and the relative position of the lower teeth is classified as Class I, II or III. Angle's Class I occlusion denotes a normal anteroposterior relationship, a Class II malocclusion indicates that the lower dentition is displaced backwards and a Class III malocclusion indicates that the lower dentition is displaced forwards. In a Class II, the overjet is usually increased, the lower canine-premolar embrasure is behind the upper canine, and the central groove of the lower molar is behind its corresponding upper landmark (see Figure 7.2). In a Class III the overbite is decreased or negative, the lower canine-premolar embrasure is in front of the upper canine, and the central grove of the lower first molar is in front of its corresponding upper landmark (see Figure 7.2).

In the vertical dimension, the occlusion is assessed by evaluating the relationship between the upper and lower teeth of the anterior and posterior dentition. The normal vertical relationship of the anterior teeth (incisors and canines) is assessed by measuring the *overbite*, which is the vertical overlap of the edges of the central incisors, measured in millimeters (see Figure 7.2). The mean normal overbite is 2 mm. In the posterior dentition (premolars and molars), a normal vertical relationship occurs when the upper and lower teeth make contact on biting. Malocclusions characterized by abnormal vertical relationships are of two types: open bites and deep bites. Both types of malocclusions can occur in the anterior teeth. However, only open bites can exist in the posterior region. Open bites can be classified by location into anterior or posterior. An anterior open bite occurs when the incisal overbite is less than zero while a posterior open bite occurs when the upper and lower premolars and molars do not make contact during biting. A deep bite occurs when the incisal overbite is greater than 4 mm.

In the transverse dimension, the occlusion is assessed by evaluating the mediolateral relationship of the upper and lower molars, premolars, and canines. A normal relationship occurs when the outer (buccal) cusps of the upper molars are positioned lateral to the buccal cusps of the lower. Malocclusions characterized by abnormal transverse relationships create cross-bites. A cross-bite occurs when the upper buccal cusps are medial to the buccal cusps of the lower molars.

The presence of malocclusion can provide important clues to the etiology of OSA in a particular patient. During the physical examination, we recommend assessing the occlusion in three dimensions (anteroposterior, vertical, and transverse). In the anteroposterior dimension, the occlusion should be classified as Class I, II or III. The majority of Class II malocclusions are caused by mandibular retrognathia, which is associated with a decreased retroglossal space.[11]

> ### ✋ CAUTION
>
> Don't be fooled by weight. Although the severity of OSA is frequently associated with obesity, a thin patient may also have severe OSA secondary to airway collapse in all the same areas.

Most Class III malocclusions are the result of mandibular prognathism, a condition that is usually not associated with OSA. However, we should keep in mind that a Class III malocclusion can also occur in midface hypoplasia, a condition associated with decreased nasopharyngeal and retropalatal airway. Finally, although a Class I occlusion is considered normal, its presence does not rule out a skeletal deformity. We should bear in mind that Angle's classification only records the *relative* position of one jaw to the other and that it is possible to have a normal Class I relationship when both jaws are retruded. Actually, this last condition is what is seen in most patients with OSA.[12] In the vertical dimension, we assess the overbite. Most open bites are the result of nasopharyngeal or oropharyngeal obstruction due to adenotonsillar hyperplasia during childhood. It is hypothesized that obstruction of nasal breathing forces patients to open the mouth, protrude the tongue, and breathe orally. Because the anterior tongue is, at all times, located between the upper and lower incisors, these teeth cannot grow towards each other. At the same time, because the mouth is always open, the posterior teeth overerupt.[13]

The final assessment of the occlusion is in the transverse dimension. Most cross-bites are the result of transverse maxillary hypoplasia or widening of the mandibular dental arch. Transverse maxillary hypoplasia is associated with a pattern of oral breathing and may reflect a narrow nasal cavity or nasopharyngeal obstruction.[14,15] Widening of the mandibular dental arch may be a sign of macroglossia (acquired or congenital).

A useful screening tool for predicting the presence of OSA is the Friedman staging system in which the examiner gives patients values based on FTP, Body Mass Index (BMI), and tonsil size (Table 7.1). The values are summed to calculate a sleep-disordered breathing (SDB) score: SDB score = FTP (0–4) + tonsil size (0–4) + BMI value (0–4). An SDB score above 8 is considered positive and has a positive predictive

Table 7.1 Friedman staging system

Grade	BMI (kg/m²)	Tonsil size
0	<20	No tonsils (post tonsillectomy)
I	20–25	Tonsils within pillars
II	25–30	Tonsils extend to pillars
III	30–40	Tonsils extend past pillars
IV	>40	Tonsils extend to midline

value of 90% for moderate OSA (Apnea Hypopnea Index [AHI] >20). A value below 4 is considered negative and is 67% effective in predicting an AHI <20.[10]

Ancillary studies

Nasopharyngoscopy

Flexible nasopharyngoscopy allows assessment of the retropalatal and retrolingual regions, two major sites of obstruction. The Müeller maneuver is a helpful flexible nasopharyngoscopic technique for identifying obstruction at the level of the palate. With a fiberoptic scope sequentially viewing the upper and lower pharynx, the supine patient is instructed to inspire with mouth closed and with nostrils occluded by the examiner. Collapse during the negative inspiratory pressure is speculated to reflect collapse during sleep. Unfortunately, the Müeller maneuver is much less useful in evaluating tongue base obstruction, since tongue base position varies with patient positioning. In addition, an awake fiberoptic laryngoscopic exam will be starkly different from one in which the patient is asleep.[16]

It is hard to predict which patients are likely to have a successful surgical outcome. Part of the reason is the difficulty associated with accurately identifying the site(s) of obstruction. Sleep endoscopy, a relatively new technique, helps define this better. Patients are examined in a drug-induced sleep-resembling relaxed state. As the patient snores and obstructs while sleeping, a flexible fiberoptic scope is passed through the nose to evaluate the upper airway to reveal the site of obstruction. This enables the surgeon to adequately address the site of obstruction while preserving areas that are not involved. The data on the validity of this procedure are scant yet promising, but this procedure may not be widely available in all areas.

Radiographic cephalometry

Radiographic cephalometry refers to the analysis of facial form done on a cephalogram. Cephalograms are plain radiographs of the face and cranium taken at a constant distance from the subject while the subject's head is stabilized in a cephalostat.[17,18] Cephalograms can be obtained in the lateral and frontal views. A lateral view is obtained with the film parallel to the sagittal plane of the patient (Figure 7.3a).

Lateral cephalograms have been utilized to evaluate patients with OSA because they facilitate the quantitative assessment of the pharyngeal airway space, the craniofacial skeleton and the visceral soft tissues. Many studies have compared the cephalometric features of OSA patients with normal controls and demonstrated significant differences between the two groups. Cephalometric studies provide evidence that, in the midsagittal plane, the pharyngeal airway is narrower in patients with OSA. This difference occurs at all levels – the nasopharynx, the oropharynx and hypopharynx.[19–22] In addition, these studies also demonstrate statistical differences in facial form between the two groups. The most significant differences relate to the mandible. Specifically, in OSA patients the body of the mandible seems to be shorter and the inferior border of the mandible seems to be steeper. Moreover, in these patients, the distance between the hyoid bone and the inferior border of the mandible is also increased.[23]

In clinical practice, the information gathered from a lateral cephalometric analysis can guide therapeutic interventions. Cephalometry is used to quantify the severity of the airway narrowing, to facilitate the determination of the site of obstruction and to help identify the etiology of the condition. At minimum, a cephalometric analysis for OSA should assess the anteroposterior dimension of the airway space at the retropalatal and retroglossal levels, the length of the soft palate, the distance from the hyoid bone to the inferior border of the mandible, and the form of the craniofacial skeleton. The determination of craniofacial form should include separate assessments of the cranial base (size and shape) and the jaws (size, shape, position, and orientation) (Figure 7.3b).

Dynamic magnetic resonance imaging

Dynamic magnetic resonance imaging (MRI) is a technique that aims to evaluate the functional narrowing of the upper airway of patients during sleep in order to determine the exact site or sites of obstruction. Patients with OSA have been shown to have significantly narrower airway diameter in the epi-, meso- and hypopharynx in sleep than in wakefulness. In comparing patients with and without OSA, patients with OSA were noted to have a more circular-shaped pharynx compared with BMI and age-matched controls. However, due to lack of clinical data and costliness, dynamic MRI is not a standard practice in the work-up of OSA patients today.[24, 25]

Surgical treatment

> ★ **TIPS AND TRICKS**
>
> Obstructive sleep apnea patients most likely to benefit from surgical therapy are those with large 4+ (kissing) tonsils.

Surgical treatment of OSA depends on a multitude of different factors. Although surgical therapy is usually reserved for those patients who have failed positive pressure therapy, there is a select subgroup of patients who may benefit from surgery first. For instance, patients with a severe nasoseptal deviation and large kissing tonsils may benefit from surgical correction first. Pediatric patients with OSA typically achieve a greater than 90% cure rate from surgical treatment of their tonsils and adenoids.[26] Patients with obvious craniofacial abnormalities may find a surgical evaluation useful as part of a formal sleep evaluation. Patients who are frequent travelers to regions without stable electricity and/or severely claustrophobic patients should also be considered initial surgical candidates. Lastly, studies have shown that compliance rates for CPAP use in teens and young adults are much poorer than in the older adult patient.[27]

Unfortunately, there exists significant variability in the current medical literature on the best treatment of OSA. This is due to different surgical techniques, combined surgical treatment of different areas, and the inherent variability of identifying the site of obstruction in patients with OSA. As a result, no universal algorithm exists. Our algorithm is developed based on our belief in performing "minimally invasive surgery" by initially identifying the primary site of obstruction via a diagnostic sleep endoscopy (Figure 7.4). This enables the preservation of anatomical areas from surgical manipulation if found to be non-obstructive. Frequently, this is performed at the same time as nasal surgery.

(a)

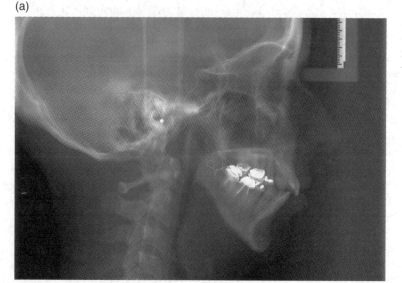

Figure 7.3 (a) Lateral cephalometric radiograph of a patient with OSAS.

(b)

LATERAL CEPHALOMETRIC ANALYSIS REPORT

CASSOS Report

Surgical plan : 03-12-2008 VTO

Patient name :
Sex :
Race :

Report time/date : 10:42 01-24-2011   Report name : OSAS analysis (Tracing)
Data source : Tracing

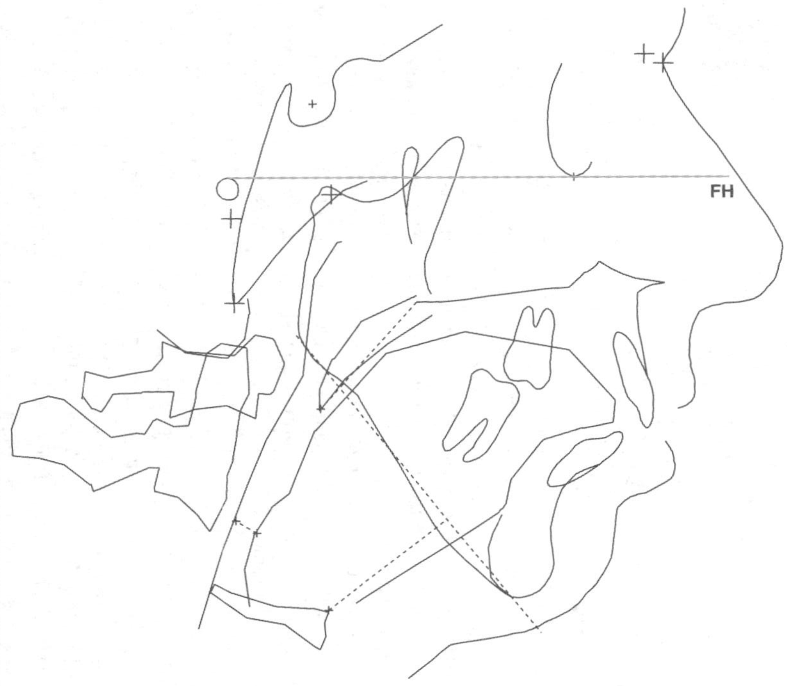

OSAS analysis

	Unit	Actual		Mean	SD
Skeleton					
1. Ar-Ptm (//HP)	mm	18.7	↓↓↓	32.8	1.9
2. Ptm-N (//HP)	mm	47.7	↓	50.9	3.0
3. Na-Sella-Ba	deg	119.6	↓↓	132.0	4.6
4. SNA	deg	79.7		80.0	3.9
5. SNB	deg	70.7	↓	78.2	3.9
6. ANB	deg	9.0		2.0	
7. Max depth	deg	88.3	↓	90.0	1.0
8. Facial angle	deg	80.0	↓↓	87.0	3.0
9. MD Plane to FH	deg	51.4	↑↑↑	26.0	4.0
10. Facial axis (XY axis)	deg	73.6	↓↓↓	90.0	3.0
Airway					
11. Soft palate length	mm	29.2		35.0	
12. Tongue to PPW	mm	4.9		11.0	
13. Hyoid to MP	mm	30.5		15.0	

FH

OSAS analysis   Horizontal plane: Frankfort plane

Mean/SD source: Unclassified\Permanent dentition\Female

Figure 7.3 (b) Cephalometric analysis.

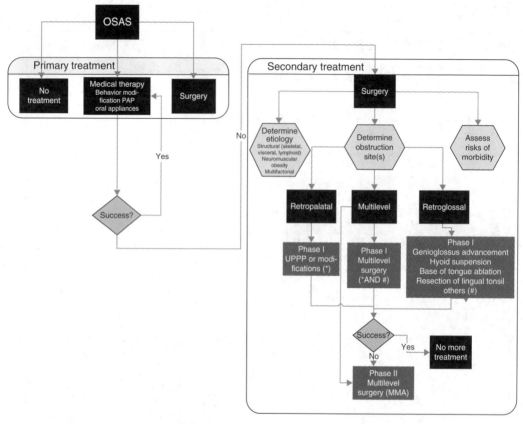

Figure 7.4 OSAS treatment algorithm.

Occasionally, the primary site of obstruction can obscure visualization of another site of obstruction. In this situation, only the primary site would be addressed, being aware that a secondary procedure involving a repeat sleep endoscopy may be required. Nasal surgery and oropharyngeal surgery are rarely performed together due to the pain involved. Nasal surgery temporarily causes nasal congestion for up to a week, resulting in pure mouth breathing which can lead to oral dryness and further discomfort. Frequently, nasal congestion and a dry, inflamed oropharynx can also cause a sense of claustrophobia in patients, making postoperative recovery that much more difficult. Separating the nasal and oropharyngeal surgeries enables better counseling of the patient regarding the findings of the sleep endoscopy and the resulting surgical plan.

If after the nasal procedure, the patient is still unable to utilize positive pressure, then the results of the sleep endoscopy are reviewed with the patient

and oropharyngeal surgery is then scheduled. If only soft palate obstruction is seen, a variation of an uvulopalatopharyngoplasty (focusing on the mid soft palate or lateral pharyngeal walls, depending on pathology) and tonsillectomy would be performed. If prominent lingual tonsils are seen, a lingual tonsillectomy would be performed. If an isolated epiglottic collapse along the posterior oropharynx is seen, a hyoid myotomy and suspension or an epiglottopexy would be appropriate. If the base of tongue and the epiglottis are both collapsing, then a hyoid myotomy and suspension would be considered, along with a partial posterior glossectomy and a genioglossal advancement. Any combination of the above may be performed depending on the findings of the sleep endoscopy. A repeat sleep study is ordered in 3 months, to allow swelling to recede and tissues to scar.

If OSA still persists then the patient has the option of repeating a diagnostic sleep endoscopy along with further "touch-up" surgery to tighten any other sites of obstruction. Depending on the patient, maxillomandibular advancement may be recommended at that time. Descriptions of the above procedures are discussed in further detail below.

In-office minor procedures

Office-based procedures are typically used in patients with the main complaint of snoring or very mild OSA. Success rates for the in-office cure of snoring are quite high, up to 80% or higher, while the in-office success rate for the cure of OSA is poor. Soft palate stents, which are intended to stiffen the soft palate and thereby decrease snoring and respiratory events, have been approved by the FDA for the treatment of snoring and mild OSA. They are only used when the cause of the OSA is secondary to a floppy but normal-length soft palate. Radiofrequency ablation of the soft palate, inferior turbinates and base of tongue are in-office procedures performed under local anesthesia. The intent is to alter the stiffness of the site of interest so that it becomes dynamically stable (palate) or decreases in size (turbinates and base of tongue). Usually, these procedures are performed to decrease upper airway resistance in patients who require high positive airway pressure therapy. By decreasing upper airway resistance, frequently the PAP pressures can be decreased, thus potentially improving machine usage compliance (i.e. decreased mask air leakage, decreased gastric air). Patients with an elongated or obstructing uvula may benefit from partial uvulectomy, a procedure easily performed in clinic. Laser-assisted uvulopalatoplasty (LAUP) is an office-based procedure used to treat snoring and mild sleep apnea. LAUP aims to reduce redundant soft tissue of the soft palate and uvula. Many patients require repeat sessions, and due to the pain involved, it is a procedure that is starting to lose favor.

Surgical procedures

Tonsillectomy and adenoidectomy

Adenotonsillectomy is the most common procedure performed to address OSA in children and has a high surgical success rate. Adults are less likely to exhibit an obstructive amount of adenoid tissue, as the adenoids begin to atrophy around the age of 8 years. However, tonsil sizes vary across the adult population. In patients with large 4+ tonsils, studies have shown that posttonsillectomy AHI improved by at least 50% in 70% of adult patients with severe OSA and 100% of those with mild-to-moderate OSA. Taking into account the site of obstruction, a tonsillectomy with or without adenoidectomy may effectively open the upper airway in select patients with site-specific obstruction. Postoperative bleeding occurs in 1–2% of patients and is the main risk factor, occurring anywhere from day 1 to day 10. Late-onset bleeding is thought to be due to the dissolution of clots on the tonsillar fossa potentially exposing an incompletely healed artery.

Nasal surgery

Nasal pathologies that lead to OSA are often addressed surgically. These pathologies include septal deviation, turbinate hypertrophy, nasal valve collapse, and obstructing nasal polyps. Nasal valve collapse (alar collapse that occurs when the patient breathes in forcefully) may be corrected with alar baton grafts to help provide cartilaginous support to weak nasal ala. Septal deviation may lead to collapse of the internal nasal valve, which is the angle created by the articulation of the upper lateral cartilages with the septum, ideally 15°. Septal deviation is corrected with a septoplasty procedure; this involves removal of obstructing bony or cartilaginous spurs, removal of the involved septum, morselization of septal cartilage and replacement of the straightened cartilage to reconstitute and straighten the septum. A nasal septal perforation, or a hole in the septum, is the main potential complication associated with a septoplasty and occurs less than 1% of the time. Enlarged inferior turbinates can be surgically reduced with partial reduction of the inferior turbinates (PRITS). Finally, obstructing polyps that do not respond to intranasal steroid therapy may be surgically removed with endoscopic sinus surgery and nasal polypectomy.

Nasal surgery is used to improve CPAP efficiency and tolerance by decreasing negative pressure breathing. Seldom does nasal surgery alone completely resolve OSA.

Uvulopalatopharyngoplasty

Retropalatal obstruction is a common site of obstruction in OSA; however, it is not commonly the only site of obstruction. Treatment of this anatomical obstruction may be addressed with a uvulopalatopharyngoplasty (UPPP). The tissue at this level is extremely compliant, exacerbating collapsibility of the retropalatal region. Dr Shiro Fujita first described UPPP in 1981, a procedure that involves tonsillectomy, trimming of the posterior and anterior tonsillar pillars, and partial excision of the uvula and soft palate.[28] UPPP or a variant of the procedure is the best way to address obstruction in patients with obstruction at the retropalatal level (occurs in 30–40% of patients with OSA). The overall success of UPPP varies from 16% to 90%. The success rate of UPPP is quite good when there is little or no obstruction retrolingually, with a cure rate of 80–90%. The success rate of a UPPP alone falls to 5–30% in patients with base of tongue involvement.[29] Velopharyngeal insufficiency is the main complication of this procedure and varies by surgical technique and surgical experience.

Lingual tonsillectomy/partial glossectomy

Retrolingual obstruction can be a challenging problem in sleep surgery. The cause of obstruction is often hypertrophic lingual tonsils, large tongue base, retroflexed epiglottis, and/or redundant supraglottic tissue. Patients with hypertrophic lingual tonsils (tonsillar tissue located at the base of tongue) causing retrolingual obstruction may undergo a lingual tonsillectomy. Macroglossia or base of tongue obstruction leading to OSA may be addressed with a partial glossectomy. Both procedures are now performed under direct visualization utilizing the DaVinci surgical robot. The partial glossectomy also entails mapping out the neurovascular bundle of the tongue using a hand-held Doppler. This prevents injury to those structures while debulking a large portion of the base of tongue. Typically, no significant voice changes or dysgeusia result from these procedures.

Hyoid myotomy and suspension

Hyoid suspension is a procedure that enlarges the retrolingual space, as the epiglottis and base of the tongue are partially attached to this skeletal structure. This procedure involves a superficial neck skin incision, isolating the hyoid bone, placing two sutures on each side of the hyoid and suspending it to the posterior inferior surface of the mandible. A neck hematoma is the primary complication associated with this surgical technique.

Genioglossus advancement

Genioglossus advancement (GA) is an operation designed to advance the anterior insertion of the genioglossi muscles. It was first introduced by Riley et al.[30] Their original technique involved a full-thickness rectangular osteotomy of the anterior mandible encompassing the location of the genial tubercles. The bony flap containing the genial tubercles and attached genioglossi muscles is pulled anteriorly and rotated until the lingual cortex of the rectangle is on top of the labial cortex of the surrounding mandible. The protruding outer cortex and marrow are removed and the remaining lingual plate is rigidly fixed to the mandible with a screw (Figure 7.5). The rationale of this operation is that by increasing the tension of the genioglossus muscle at rest, the collapse of the tongue base into the airway, as it occurs in hypotonia, is prevented.

Because of technical difficulties with the original technique, several surgeons have developed alternative procedures. Some of the most popular variations include the genial bone advancement trephine (GBAT),[31,32] the two-piece GA with trapezoidal bone flap,[24] and a high genioplasty incorporating the genial tubercles.[33,34] This operation is almost always done in conjunction with other procedures as part of the multilevel treatment of sleep apnea; because of this, the effectiveness if this operation has not been determined. Possible complications from this operation include sensory disturbance in the lower lip and chin, hematoma formation in the floor of the mouth, infection, accidental tear or detachment of the genioglossi muscles, iatrogenic injury to the roots of the lower incisors and canines, and pathological fracture of the mandible. However, in our experience the rate of complications has been very low.

Maxillomandibular advancement

Maxillomandibular advancement (MMA) is an operation that moves the maxilla and mandible forwards to increase the airway size. The magnitude of the jaw advancement is typically in the order of 10–12 mm. In most centers, the operation begins in the upper jaw. In the first step, the maxilla is separated from the midface skeleton by completing a horizontal osteotomy above the level of the nasal floor (LeFort I osteotomy). The soft and hard palate remained attached to the maxilla to provide vascularity to the bony segment. After the maxilla has been freed from its bony attachments, it is moved forwards and rigidly fixed in the new position using four titanium miniplates. Since the soft palate is

(a)

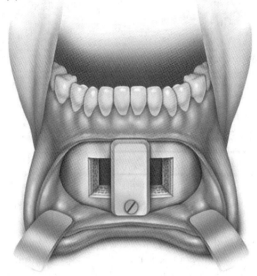

(b)

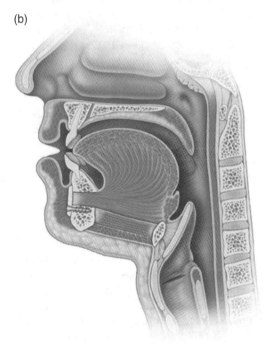

Figure 7.5 Genioglossus advancement. (a) Front view. (b) Lateral view.

attached to the maxilla, the forward movement of the latter results in advancement of the soft palate and enlargement of the retropalatal airway space.

In the second part of the operation, the mandible is advanced. This is accomplished by first completing sagittal osteotomies of the mandibular rami. The sagittal osteotomies divide the mandible into two proximal segments (right and left) and a distal segment. The proximal segments contain the mandibular condyles, the outer cortex of the rami, and the outer cortex of the posterior body. The distal segment contains the whole dentition, the remainder of the body of the mandible, and the inner cortex of the rami. Once the osteotomies have been completed, the distal segment is advanced until the lower teeth achieve normal dental interdigitation (occlusion) with the upper. Once in this position, the proximal segments are rigidly fixed to the distal segment using miniplates and/or screws. Since the tongue is attached to the distal mandible at the genial tubercles, advancement of the mandible produces advancement of the tongue and an increase of the retroglossal airway space. Advancement of the genial tubercles also results in stretching of the geniohyoid muscle with consequent hyoid advancement (Figure 7.6).

Because of its magnitude, MMA is usually reserved for patients with moderate and severe OSA who have failed medical treatment (e.g. PAP) and phase I multilevel surgery. However, in selected patients, MMA may be the best option for primary treatment. Included in the last group are patients with concomitant jaw deformities that require the same surgical procedures for treatment. MMA is contraindicated in patients with significant risks of perioperative morbidity and mortality due to co-morbid medical conditions.

With the exception of a tracheostomy, MMA is the most effective operation for the treatment of OSA in adults. A recent metaanalysis of 627 patients who underwent MMA for the treatment of OSA reports significant improvements from surgery. Overall, the AHI decreased from 63.9 ± 26.7/hour to 9.5 ± 10.7/hour, the SpO_2 nadir increased from 71.9% to 87.7%, and the Epworth scores decreased from 13.2 ± 5.5 to 5.1 ± 3.6. Using an endpoint of an AHI <5, the cure rate was reported as 43.2%. However, the outcomes of the majority of patients who did not obtained a cure should not be considered failures since even in these patients, the differences between the preoperative and postoperative indices were statistically and clinically significant (preoperative AHI of 68.3 ± 27.5/hour and postoperative AHI of 15.9 ± 1.5/hour, $p<0.001$).[35]

When considering success, it is important to remember that this operation is usually done in patients who have failed PAP and phase I multilevel

Maxillomandibular advancement

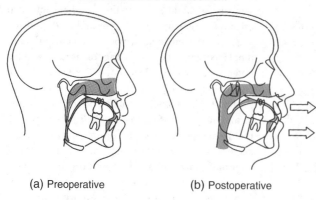

(a) Preoperative   (b) Postoperative

Figure 7.6 Maxillomandibular advancement.

surgery, thus their only remaining options are no treatment or tracheostomy. Since the mortality adjusted hazard ratios for patients with untreated OSAS are 1.4, 1.7 and 3.8 for mild, moderate and severe disease (p-trend=0.004),[36] decreasing the severity of the condition from severe to mild should positively impact mortality. The same can also be said about the quality of life since the postoperative ESS of those patients who were not cured was 6.3±2.1, a significant reduction from baseline of 13.2±5.5 (p<0.0001).[35]

Based on these analyses, leading investigators have recommended the appraisal of the effectiveness of this operation using two different endpoints. One is *surgical cure* defined as postoperative AHI <5 and the other *surgical success* defined as postoperative AHI <20 and a ≥50% reduction in AHI. Using the last endpoint, success rate of this operation has been estimated to be 86.0%.[35]

Finally, there is a widespread belief that this operation is associated with significant morbidity. However, data from a recent metaanalysis of MMA outcomes does not support this contention.[35] In this analysis, the rate of major complications was 1% and the minor complication rate was 3.1%. The major complications were mostly cardiac events and the majority of minor complications were malocclusions (44%) and sensory disturbances of the face (14%). No deaths were reported.

Tracheostomy

In severe forms of OSA, a tracheostomy is curative in completely bypassing the upper airway and eliminating sleep apnea. Patients who typically fall within this category either have severe craniofacial abnormalities or are morbidly obese. Performing a tracheostomy in a morbidly obese patient is associated with a higher risk of surgical complications, is technically much more difficult to accomplish, and the morbidities associated with the procedure, including wound care issues, must be considered.

Follow-up

For patients who undergo surgery, retesting is indicated. The interval at which retesting should be done depends on the type of surgery that was performed. Retesting 3 months following the surgical intervention is adequate in most cases.

Conclusion

Surgical treatment for patients with sleep-disordered breathing is an important management option, particularly in those patients with specific physical examination findings or for those who have not tolerated CPAP. Nasal surgery may initially be performed in order to decrease CPAP settings and improve CPAP compliance. Physical examination and endoscopy may help assess the optimal surgical options for some patients. In most cases, staged surgery, starting with less invasive procedures and if necessary performing more invasive surgeries, is a preferred approach.

References

1. Al Lawati NM, Patel SR, Ayas NT. Epidemiology, risk factors, and consequences of obstructive sleep apnea and short sleep duration. *Progr Cardiovasc Dis* 2009; **51**(4): 285–93.

2. Punjabi NM. The epidemiology of adult obstructive sleep apnea. *Proc Am Thorac Soc* 2008; **5**(2): 136–43.

3. Ancoli-Israel S, Klauber MR, Stepnowsky C, Estline E, Chinn A, Fell R. Sleep-disordered breathing in African-American elderly. *Am J Respir Crit Care Med* 1995; **152**(6 Pt 1): 1946–9.

4. Institute for Clinical Systems Improvement. *I. Diagnosis and Treatment of Obstructive Sleep Apnea in Adults*. Bloomington, MN: Institute for Clinical Systems Improvement, 2008.

5. Gottlieb DJ, Whitney CW, Bonekat WH, et al. Relation of sleepiness to respiratory disturbance index: the Sleep Heart Health Study. *Am J Respir Crit Care Med* 1999; **159**(2): 502–7.

6. Li KK, Powell NB, Kushida C, Riley RW, Adornato B, Guilleminault C. A comparison of Asian and white patients with obstructive sleep apnea syndrome. *Laryngoscope* 1999; **109**(12): 1937–40.

7. Peppard PE, Young T, Palta M, Dempsey J, Skatrud J. Longitudinal study of moderate weight change and sleep-disordered breathing. *JAMA* 2000; **284**(23): 3015–21.

8. Quan SF, Howard BV, Iber C, et al. The Sleep Heart Health Study: design, rationale, and methods. *Sleep* 1997; **20**(12): 1077–85.

9. Giles TL, Lasserson TJ, Smith BH, White J, Wright J, Cates CJ. Continuous positive airways pressure for obstructive sleep apnoea in adults. *Cochrane Database Syst Rev* 2006; **3**: CD001106.

10. Friedman M, Soans R, Gurpinar B, Lin H, Joseph N. Interexaminer agreement of Friedman tongue positions for staging of obstructive sleep apnea/hypopnea syndrome. *Otolaryngol Head Neck Surg* 2008; **139**: 372–7.

11. Miyao E, Noda A, Miyao M, Yasuma F, Inafuku S. The role of malocclusion in non-obese patients with obstructive sleep apnea syndrome. *Intern Med* 2008; **47**(18): 1573–8.

12. Bacon WH, Krieger J, Turlot JC, Stierle JL. Craniofacial characteristics in patients with obstructive sleep apneas syndrome. *Cleft Palate J* 1988; **25**(4): 374–8.

13. Leighton BC. Aetiology of malocclusion of the teeth. *Arch Dis Child* 1991; **66**(9): 1011–12.

14. Ramires T, Maia RA, Barone JR. Nasal cavity changes and the respiratory standard after maxillary expansion. *Braz J Otorhinolaryngol* 2008; **74**(5): 763–9.

15. Villa MP, Malagola C, Pagani J, et al. Rapid maxillary expansion in children with obstructive sleep apnea syndrome: 12-month follow-up. *Sleep Med* 2007; **8**(2): 128–34.

16. Sher AE, Thorpy MJ, Shprintzen RJ, Spielman AJ, Burack B, McGregor PA. Predictive value of Muller maneuver in selection of patients for uvulopalatopharyngoplasty. *Laryngoscope* 1985; **95**(12): 1483–7.

17. Broadbent BH. A new X-ray technique and its application to orthodontia: the introduction of cephalometric radiography. *Angle Orthod* 1931; **1**(1): 45–66.

18. Broadbent BH, BroadbentBH JR, Golden WH. *Bolton Standards of Dentofacial Development Growth*. St Louis, MO: V.V. Mosby, 1975.

19. Lyberg T, Krogstad O, Djupesland G. Cephalometric analysis in patients with obstructive sleep apnoea syndrome. I. Skeletal morphology. *J Laryngol Otol* 1989; **103**(3): 287–92.

20. Lyberg T, Krogstad O, Djupesland G. Cephalometric analysis in patients with obstructive sleep apnoea syndrome: II. Soft tissue morphology. *J Laryngol Otol* 1989; **103**(3): 293–7.

21. deBerry-Borowiecki B, Kukwa A, Blanks RH. Cephalometric analysis for diagnosis and treatment of obstructive sleep apnea. *Laryngoscope* 1988; **98**(2): 226–34.

22. Strelzow VV, Blanks RH, Basile A, Strelzow AE. Cephalometric airway analysis in obstructive sleep apnea syndrome. *Laryngoscope* 1988; **98**(11): 1149–58.

23. Miles PG, Vig PS, Weyant RJ, Forrest TD, Rockette HE Jr. Craniofacial structure and obstructive sleep apnea syndrome – a qualitative analysis and meta-analysis of the literature. *Am J Orthod Dentofacial Orthop* 1996; **109**(2): 163–72.

24. Ciscar MA, Juan G, Martinez V, et al. Magnetic resonance imaging of the pharynx in OSA patients and healthy subjects. *Eur Respir J* 2001; **17**(1): 79–86.

25. Shintani T, Kozawa T, Himi T. Obstructive sleep apnea by analysis of MRI findings. *International Congress Series* 2003; **1257**: 99–102.

26. Nakata S, Noda A, Yanagi E. Results of tonsillectomy for obstructive sleep apnea syndrome in adults with tonsillar hypertrophy. *International Congress Series* 2003; **1257**: 95–8.

27. Sher AE, Schechtman KB, Piccirillo JF. The efficacy of surgical modifications of the upper airway in adults with obstructive sleep apnea syndrome. *Sleep* 1996; **19**(2): 156–77.

28. Fujita S, Conway W, Zorick F, Roth T. Surgical correction of anatomic abnormalities in obstructive sleep apnea syndrome: uvulopalatopharyngoplasty. *Otolaryngol Head Neck Surg* 1981; **89**(6): 923–34.

29. Khan A, Ramar K, Maddirala S, Friedman O, Pallanch JF, Olson EJ. Uvulopalatopharyngoplasty in the management of obstructive sleep apnea: the Mayo Clinic experience. *Mayo Clin Proc* 2009; **84**(9): 795–800.

30. Riley RW, Powell NB, Guilleminault C. Inferior mandibular osteotomy and hyoid myotomy suspension for obstructive sleep apnea: a review of 55 patients. *J Oral Maxillofac Surg* 1989; **47**(2): 159–64.

31. Hennessee J, Miller FR. Anatomic analysis of the genial bone advancement trephine system's effectiveness at capturing the genial tubercle and its muscular attachments. *Otolaryngol Head Neck Surg* 2005; **133**(2): 229–33.

32. Lewis MR, Ducic Y. Genioglossus muscle advancement with the genioglossus bone advancement technique for base of tongue obstruction. *J Otolaryngol* 2003; **32**(3): 168–73.

33. Lee NR, Madani M. Genioglossus muscle advancement techniques for obstructive sleep apnea. *Atlas Oral Maxillofac Surg Clin North Am* 2007; **15**(2): 179–92.

34. Hendler B, Silverstein K, Giannakopoulos H, Costello BJ. Mortised genioplasty in the treatment of obstructive sleep apnea: an historical perspective and modification of design. *Sleep Breathing (Schlaf & Atmung)* 2001; **5**(4): 173–80.

35. Holty JE, Guilleminault C. Maxillomandibular advancement for the treatment of obstructive sleep apnea: a systematic review and meta-analysis. *Sleep Med Rev* 2010; **14**(5): 287–97.

36. Young T, Finn L, Peppard PE, et al. Sleep disordered breathing and mortality: eighteen-year follow-up of the Wisconsin sleep cohort. *Sleep* 2008; **31**(8): 1071–8.

8

Medical Co-morbidities Associated with Obstructive Sleep Apnea

Emerson M. Wickwire, PhD[1,2] and Scott G. Williams, MD[3]

[1] Pulmonary Disease and Critical Care Associates, USA
[2] Department of Psychiatry and Behavioral Sciences, Johns Hopkins School of Medicine, USA
[3] Department of Pulmonary, Critical Care and Sleep Medicine, Womack Army Medical Center, USA

Introduction

Obstructive sleep apnea (OSA) is associated with a number of short-term and long-term adverse health consequences. Further, the symptoms of OSA can easily be mistaken for other medical or psychiatric conditions. It is thus especially important for healthcare professionals across disciplines to be familiar with not only the consequences but also the often subtle presentations of OSA. The purpose of this chapter is to review the medical co-morbidities of OSA but it is not intended to serve as an exhaustive review. Rather, we seek to provide an overview of the most germane findings pertaining to the medical consequences of OSA, with an eye to real-world application. We review the implications of the most robust findings in seven key domains: mortality, cardiovascular disease, cerebrovascular events, endocrine dysfunction, neurocognitive dysfunction, psychiatric co-morbidity, and other sleep disorders. Because it remains the most commonly prescribed and considered most effective treatment for OSA, we also review the effect of treatment with positive airway pressure (PAP) on these consequences of OSA. Readers are referred to other chapters in this volume to learn more about alternative treatment approaches. Clinical recommendations are included throughout the chapter.

Mortality

The association between OSA and all-cause mortality has been demonstrated in both cross-sectional and prospective reports. Marshall et al. analyzed 14-year follow-up data from 380 community residents of Busselton, Australia, who underwent home sleep testing for OSA at baseline.[1] In this study moderate-to-severe OSA (but not mild OSA) was associated with greater risk of all-cause mortality than was non-OSA even after controlling for age, gender, Body Mass Index (BMI), blood pressure, cholesterol, diabetes, and angina (hazard ratio = 6.24). Similarly, Punjabi et al. performed a prospective analysis of 8.2-year follow-up data of middle-aged men and women participating in the Sleep Heart Health Study (n = 6441).[2] After controlling for age, sex, ethnicity, smoking, BMI, and medical co-morbidities, severe OSA (Apnea Hypopnea Index [AHI] ≥30) was significantly associated with increased risk of death in men age 40–70 (hazard ratio = 2.09). Notably, this study also found sleep-related intermittent hypoxemia, but not sleep fragmentation, to be independently associated with all-cause mortality. Hypoxemia but not sleep fragmentation was also related to coronary artery disease-related mortality associated with OSA.[2] Similarly, a recent retrospective analysis among

Sleep Medicine in Neurology, First Edition. Edited by Douglas B. Kirsch.
© 2014 John Wiley & Sons, Ltd. Published 2014 by John Wiley & Sons, Ltd.

patients under 50 years of age found O_2 nadir during sleep to be correlated with mortality even after controlling for baseline medical co-morbidities.[3] As we review below, the increased mortality in untreated OSA is primarily due to worsened cardiovascular outcomes. Among the putative mechanisms are increased sympathetic autonomic activity from intermittent hypoxemia, oxidative stress, endothelial dysfunction and an overall increase in systemic inflammation as well as endocrine and metabolic derangements.

Treatment with PAP may reduce all-cause mortality associated with OSA. In a study of 871 patients followed for an average of 4 years, Campos-Rodriguez et al. found increased PAP use to be positively correlated with survival.[4] Relative to PAP non-adherent patients (i.e. those who used PAP ≤1 hour/nt), highly adherent patients (i.e. who used PAP ≥6 hour/nt) demonstrated significantly higher 5-year survival rates (96.4% versus 85.5%, p < 0.00005). Similarly, relative to non-adherent patients, moderately adherent patients (i.e. who used PAP from 1 hour to 6 hour/nt) also demonstrated increased cumulative 5-year survival (91.3% versus 85.5%, p = 0.01). Further, a significant trend toward increased survival across groups was identified (p = 0.0004). As is often the case, in this study cardiovascular disease (CVD) was the leading cause of death. More recently, PAP has been shown to reduce cardiovascular mortality risk in women[5] and elderly patients with AHI ≥30.[6]

---

disease. For example, in a randomized trial among minimally symptomatic OSA patients, PAP was associated with improvements in subjective and objective sleepiness as well as perceived health status, but was unrelated to 5-year calculated vascular risk.[8] It is worth noting, however, that mean PAP use was lower than traditionally considered acceptable (2 hours 39 m/nt at 6-month follow-up). Of course, prior to abandoning a prescribed course of treatment, all OSA patients should undergo thorough education and/or supplemental intervention such as cognitive-behavioral treatment or hypnotic therapy to facilitate PAP adherence.[9]

Cardiovascular consequences and co-morbidities

Systemic hypertension

Approximately 70% of OSA patients are hypertensive. Among animals, a causal relationship has been demonstrated between sleep apnea and hypertension,[10] and among humans OSA has been shown to precede the onset of hypertension. Peppard et al. conducted a prospective analysis using data from the Wisconsin Sleep Cohort.[11] Results indicated that baseline AHI was positively correlated with high blood pressure 4 years later, even after controlling for BMI, sex, waist circumference, neck circumference, alcohol consumption, and cigarette smoking. Relative to patients without sleep apnea, patients with AHI ≥15 were nearly three times more likely to develop hypertension over the 4-year follow-up period.[11] The 2003 report of the Joint National Committee on Prevention, Detection, Evaluation, and Treatment of High Blood Pressure lists sleep apnea first among secondary causes of hypertension.[12]

Treatment of OSA improves hypertension. In a study with nearly 50% of participants taking anti-hypertensive medications, Becker et al. found PAP reduced mean arterial pressure by nearly 10 mmHg (p = 0.01).[13] Similarly, Logan et al. found that among patients with OSA and refractory hypertension, PAP reduced 24-hours blood pressure by 10 mmHg systolic and 6 mmHg diastolic.[17] A metaanalysis of 16 randomized controlled trials (RCTs) (total n = 818 subjects with hypertension and OSA) found that PAP resulted in significant improvements in blood pressure.[14]

To dip or not to dip?
Patients with OSA do not demonstrate the lowering of blood pressure and heart rate that typically takes place during sleep.[15] This physiological decline is known as "dipping" and non-dippers demonstrate higher rates of stroke, more end-organ damage, and worse medical outcomes than patients who dip normally. In fact, although speculative, it is possible that non-dippers with OSA are at increased risk of death during apneic episodes. Gami et al. conducted a retrospective review of 112 patients who had undergone polysomnography (PSG) and then died unexpectedly.[16] Nearly half of the patients with OSA died between midnight and 6.00 am, whereas only 21% of patients without OSA died during the night.

Difficult-to-control hypertension
Consider OSA in any patient with hypertension, especially difficult-to-control hypertension.[17] Have a low threshold for performing overnight PSG in patients with a suggestive clinical history of sleep apnea even if there are no significant daytime symptoms. Successful treatment of OSA may lead to improved blood pressure measures and in some cases may lead to reduction in antihypertensive medication.

Pulmonary hypertension

Sleep apnea can be a secondary cause of pulmonary hypertension (PH). During apneic episodes of OSA, hypoxic vasoconstriction of the pulmonary arteries causes pulmonary pressures to increase. Longer and more severe desaturations are associated with greater increases in pulmonary pressures during the night. Most prevalence estimates of pulmonary hypertension among patients with OSA average about 20%. When OSA is the sole cause of PH, pulmonary hemodynamics are usually only mildy affected.[18] However, a recent study by Minai and colleagues did find that OSA was associated with severe PH in a minority of patients.[19]

To evaluate treatment effect on pulmonary hypertension, Arias et al. conducted an RCT (using sham PAP set at 2 cmH_2O) and found that PAP reduced the mean pulmonary systolic pressure from 29 to 24 mmHg (p < 0.0001).[20] The greatest reductions were found among patients with pulmonary hypertension or left ventricular diastolic dysfunction at baseline.

Cardiac arrhythmias

Mehra et al. analyzed data from the Sleep Heart Health Study (n = 456 matched for age, sex, race, and BMI) and found atrial fibrillation and non-sustained ventricular tachycardia (NSVT) to be higher in OSA patients (AHI ≥30) than in people without OSA (AHI <5).[21] More recently, Monahan et al. found that paroxysms of atrial fibrillation or episodes of NSVT were more likely to occur within 90 sec of an apneic or hypopneic event than during normal breathing, suggesting that sleep-related breathing poses an increased risk for arrhythmias.[22]

Obstructive sleep apnea also has significant impact on treatment for cardiac arrhythmias. Patients who remained in atrial fibrillation despite two catheter ablation procedures demonstrated significantly higher rates of OSA than patients successfully treated with one procedure.[23] Similarly, Patel et al. conducted a large (n = 3000, including 21% with OSA) multicenter study and reported that compared to patients without OSA, OSA patients had lower procedural success and more procedure-related complications.[24] Further, patients on PAP had lower atrial fibrillation recurrence rates.[24] Indeed, PAP has been found to reduce recurrence of atrial fibrillation following cardioversion (82% versus 42% successful cardioversion[25]) and reduce ventricular arrhythmias (PVCs) during sleep by 58%.[26]

Congestive heart failure

Up to 35% of patients with congestive heart failure also suffer from OSA, and treatment with PAP improves outcomes in these patients. In a randomized study among patients with systolic congestive heart failure (ejection fraction [EF] <45%) and severe OSA,

Kaneko et al. found that adding PAP to optimal medical treatment increased EF from 25% to 34% (p<0.001) and reduced systolic blood pressure by 10 mmHg (p=0.03) after 1 month of PAP therapy.[27] No changes were observed in the optimal medical treatment alone condition. Similarly, Khayat et al. found that among patients with acute heart failure and OSA, PAP improved left ventricular ejection fraction.[28] A small study of patients with chronic heart failure revealed improvement in left ventricular (LV) ejection fraction, a decrease in LV end-systolic volume, a decrease in right-sided heart volumes and an improvement in New York Heart Association (NYHA) functional status after 6 months of PAP. Of note, half of the patients used CPAP for this study and half were prescribed adaptive servoventilation (ASV) due to concomitant central apnea events.[29]

Cardiovascular disease

Prevalence estimates for OSA in patients with cardiovascular disease (CVD) range from 30% to 60% and far exceed those of the general population.[30] Among men hospitalized for acute myocardial infarction, the prevalence of OSA has been reported to approach 70%.[31] More important, OSA worsens outcomes within this population. For example, Shahar et al. found OSA to be an independent predictor of coronary artery disease even after controlling for well-known risk factors.[32] In a prospective analysis of 8-year follow-up data from the Sleep Heart Health Study, Punjabi et al. found a 70% greater risk of CVD-related death among patients with AHI ≥15 relative to those with AHI ≤5.[33] Similarly, Shah et al. found that CVD risk increased with increasing AHI, even after controlling for hypertension and BMI.

Although randomized studies are needed, evidence suggests that PAP improves outcomes in cardiovascular disease. In a 10-year longitudinal study, Marin et al. found that PAP reduced the incidence of ischemic events by 50%.[35] Further, relative to men with untreated mild or moderate OSA, snoring, or treated OSA, men with untreated severe OSA experienced a three-fold greater risk for both fatal and non-fatal cardiovascular events.[35]

Cerebrovascular disease/stroke

There is a strong and well-documented relationship between OSA and increased risk for cerebrovascular events. Among patients with acute stroke or transient ischemic attack, prevalence estimates for OSA are consistently well above 50%, and OSA worsens cerebrovascular outcomes. Shahar et al. analyzed data from the Sleep Heart Health Study and found higher AHI to be associated with greater risk of stroke even after controlling for common risk factors.[32] Similarly, Yaggi et al. found patients with AHI ≥5 to be 1.97 times more likely to suffer stroke or death from any cause than patients without OSA, even after controlling for hypertension and other variables. Redline et al. analyzed 9-year follow-up data (n >6000) and found that men with moderate-to-severe OSA were nearly three times as likely to have an incident ischemic stroke relative to men without OSA, even after controlling for age, BMI, smoking, systolic blood pressure, use of antihypertensive medications, diabetes, and race.[37]

In terms of mechanisms, recent controlled experimental data suggest that even in the absence of frank OSA, snoring might significantly increase risk for stroke by causing vibration in neck tissues, thereby inducing carotid endothelial dysfunction.[38] In addition to these experimental data, at least three OSA-related factors could cause stroke. First, when an apnea takes place, oxygen saturation drops while carbon dioxide levels increase, causing dilation of cerebral blood vessels and increasing cerebral blood flow. Second, intermittent hypoxia associated with OSA results in endothelial dysfunction and increased vascular oxidative stress. Finally, OSA is associated with elevated platelet activation and fibrinogen levels, resulting in a thrombosis-prone state.

Although patients with OSA experience worse outcomes than those without OSA,[39, 40] treatment of OSA is difficult in stroke patients. In a representative investigation, only seven of 32 stroke patients with OSA continued to use PAP after the first week of an 8-week PAP trial.[41] When treating patients with stroke, it can be especially helpful to include a caregiver or bed partner.

Endocrine consequences and co-morbidities

Both oxygen desaturation and AHI have been associated with insulin resistance and glucose intolerance even after controlling for BMI.[42, 43] In the Sleep Heart Health Study, participants underwent at-home sleep testing and both fasting and 2-hours glucose tolerance tests.[44, 45] Participants with AHI ≥5 were twice as likely to demonstrate impaired glucose tolerance, and the severity of impairment was related to degree of apneic desaturation.[45] Similarly, Reichmuth et al. analyzed data from 1387 participants in the Wisconsin Sleep Cohort.[46] At baseline, 15% of patients with AHI ≥15 had diabetes, whereas the prevalence of diabetes among patients with AHI ≤5 was 3%. At 4-year follow-up, there was a non-significant trend toward increased risk of developing diabetes (odds ratio [OR] = 1.62) with AHI ≥15 relative to AHI <5.

Obstructive sleep apnea may cause diabetes via three mechanisms. First, OSA is associated with sleep fragmentation, which results in glucose intolerance. Second, OSA is associated with reduced total sleep time, which can cause appetite dysregulation, resulting in insulin resistance and in some patients increase the risk of type 2 diabetes.[47] Third, patients with OSA also experience intermittent hypoxemia, which activates the sympathetic nervous system. This results in increased cortisol, catecholamines, ghrelin, and stress hormones, which may cause glucose intolerance, insulin resistance, and diabetes. In light of the known associations between these endocrine functions and obesity, it is important to recall that obesity increases OSA risk. Newman et al. found that a 10% increase in body weight was associated with over a 30% increase in AHI, and the risk of developing moderate or severe OSA increased six-fold.[48]

Although data are mixed, evidence suggests that treating OSA can improve metabolic function in OSA patients. A recent meta-analysis found that PAP therapy improved insulin resistance but not glycemic control in non-diabetic patients with OSA.[49] Nonetheless, the impact of PAP therapy on metabolic function remains a subject of much debate. In clinical practice, patients should be advised that PAP may help improve their diabetic control as well as appetite regulation. Although PAP therapy may be necessary to manage OSA, it is not sufficient to manage diabetes or facilitate weight loss.

Neurocognitive consequences and co-morbidities

Many clinicians are surprised to learn that global assessments of OSA and cognitive functioning have produced inconsistent results. For example, in a recent report of neuropsychological performance in the Apnea Positive Pressure Long-Term Efficacy Study (APPLES), weak correlations were detected between AHI and oxygen desaturation and measures of global neurocognitive performance. When analyses were adjusted for education, ethnicity, and gender, only severity of oxygen desaturation remained a significant predictor of select measures of intelligence, attention, and processing speed.[50] Yet these results may speak more to the need for comprehensive assessment of neurocognitive performance than to the lack of relationship between OSA and cognition. Previous studies with more targeted assessment of neurocognitive function provide insight into the impact of OSA on cognition.

Beebe et al. conducted a metaanalysis of 25 studies (total n = 1991) examining neurocognitive functioning among adults with untreated OSA and healthy controls.[51] Domains of cognitive function most frequently affected by OSA were selective attention/concentration, short-term/working memory, executive functioning, and motor functioning. Negligible impact was detected on intellectual and language functioning.[51] More recently, Mazza et al. administered extended vigilance and attention testing to 20 OSA patients.[52] Ninety-five percent of OSA patients had vigilance or attention deficits compared to controls (n = 40). Importantly, from a clinical perspective these findings suggest that OSA patients may experience impairments both in staying vigilant during monotonous tasks and in processing information in complex environments.

In part because of the complexity of the constructs, it has been difficult to measure the impact of OSA on memory and executive function. Nonetheless, evidence suggests a relationship between OSA and both domains of cognitive function. For example, Naëgelé et al. found that relative to matched controls, OSA patients demonstrated mild but significant impairment in episodic, procedural, and working memory domains.[53] From a mechanistic standpoint, compromised brain function may underlie poor performance among OSA patients on a working memory task.[54] Archbold et al. found OSA severity to be positively correlated with increased neuronal activity in the right parietal lobe but decreased in the cerebellar vermis.[55] These results suggest that OSA severity may correlate with neuronal activation during tasks of working memory. OSA also appears to impact executive function, For example, Salorio et al. found that relative to healthy matched controls, OSA patients demonstrated weaker use of semantic cues and poorer overall semantic clustering than healthy controls.[56]

Finally, psychomotor performance appears to be impaired in OSA patients. Aloia et al. conducted a review of peer-reviewed studies published between 1985 and 2002 and found that differences appeared to be related more to motor coordination than motor speed.[57] These authors note that psychomotor function does not appear to benefit from PAP therapy, suggesting possible irreversible damage to the central nervous system (CNS) in patients with severe OSA. Notably, this finding also suggests that psychomotor performance is unrelated to hypoxemia.

In general, PAP has been shown to improve cognitive performance.[57] More specifically, attention/vigilance improved in a majority of studies, global functioning, executive functioning, and memory improved in half of studies, and psychomotor function improved in few studies. A more recent investigation found improved memory function among patients who used PAP ≥ 6 hour/nt relative to those who used PAP ≥ 2 hour/nt, suggesting that in contrast to psychomotor performance optimal PAP adherence might reverse OSA-related memory deficits.[58]

Psychological co-morbidity

> **⚠ CAUTION**
>
> Obstructive sleep apnea can cause pathological levels of sleepiness, and untreated OSA has particularly strong associations with risk for motor vehicle accidents.[59] It appears this association is due to sleepiness rather than CNS damage, and a recent metaanalysis found that PAP reduced sleepiness and attendant risk for motor vehicle accidents.[60] Always advise caution while driving, particularly during the diagnostic and early treatment period. Clinicians should also exercise caution when prescribing benzodiazepines, centrally acting muscle relaxants, and opiates in untreated OSA patients or in patients at risk for OSA.

Although there is a wide variation in the prevalence of depression across the available studies, up to half of OSA patients experience depressive symptoms.[61] Further, patients with OSA appear to experience elevated rates of numerous psychiatric conditions. For example, Sharafkhaneh et al. reviewed over 4 million records from the centralized VA healthcare database and estimated a prevalence of OSA of 2.91%.[62] Of those with OSA, the most common psychiatric diagnoses were depression (21.8%), anxiety (16.7%), posttraumatic stress disorder (11.9%), psychosis (5.1), and bipolar disorder (3.3%). Relative to patients without OSA, those with OSA demonstrated significantly higher rates of mood disorders, anxiety, posttraumatic stress disorder, psychosis, and dementia (all statistically significant). Patients with serious mental illness (SMI) such as schizophrenia may also demonstrate increased rates of OSA. For example, 69% of patients with SMI in a primary care setting screened as high risk for OSA even though only 16% had been previously diagnosed.[63] Most patients reported that OSA had never been discussed with them, and importantly 71% were willing to be referred for a sleep evaluation if their provider recommended it.

In a large-scale study, Ohayon analyzed data from 18,980 randomly selected telephone survey participants in four Western European countries.[64] Ages ranged from 15 to 100 years. Using DSM-IV criteria, 2.1% of the sample reported symptoms consistent with OSA, and an additional 2.5% reported symptoms consistent with another DSM-IV sleep-related breathing disorder. Nearly 18% of participants meeting criteria for depression also met criteria for OSA, and 17.6% of participants reporting symptoms consistent with a sleep-related breathing disorder also met criteria for major depressive disorder.[64] Even after controlling for obesity and hypertension, participants with major depression were found to be 5.26 times more likely to develop OSA than were non-depressed participants. As these results suggest, the relationship between depression and OSA could be bidirectional. Although data are lacking, the mechanistic link between depression and OSA may be decreased upper airway dilator tone.

In terms of physiological mechanisms, the severity of depression and anxiety has been correlated with the level of nocturnal hypoxemia, severity of OSA, degree of sleep fragmentation and degree of daytime somnolence. Indeed, daytime somnolence has been shown to be one of the more powerful predictors of depressive symptoms.[65] Further, patients with OSA and depression may have different neural functioning when compared with non-depressed

OSA patients or healthy controls. Intermittent hypoxia is thought to damage the mid and anterior cingulate, anterior insular, medial prefrontal, parietal, and left ventrolateral temporal cortices, left caudate nucleus, and internal capsule. Further, relative to asymptomatic non-OSA controls, depressed OSA patients showed damage in the bilateral hippocampus, caudate, anterior corpus callosum, right anterior thalamus, and medial pons. A number of these areas are correlated with anhedonia and other negative symptoms of depression.[66]

When patients present with both a mood disorder and OSA, treatment sequence should be based on symptom severity. For example, when treating patients with mild depressive symptoms, clinicians should consider targeting OSA first. If successful treatment of OSA does not alleviate the mood distrubance, or if mood disorders affect adherence, then clinicians should consider psychotherapy or psychopharmacotherapy. Conversely, when patients present with moderate psychiatric symptoms, it may be most appropriate to treat both conditions concurrently. In severe cases, it may be necessary to stabilize psychiatric symptoms prior to initiating PAP or other OSA therapy. Of course, if there are patient safety issues at any time, emergenct medication may be required.

Decreased quality of life

Using data from the Wisconsin Sleep Cohort, Finn et al. performed in-lab PSG on 737 middle-aged adults (421 men and 316 women) enrolled in the Wisconsin Sleep Cohort Study.[67] Quality of life was assessed using interview and the SF-36, a well-validated and frequently employed self-report measure of general health and life satisfaction. After controlling for age, sex, BMI, smoking, alcohol usage, and heart disease, even mild OSA (AHI ≥ 5) was associated with lower quality of life in multiple domains. Degree of impairment was comparable to chronic medical conditions such as arthritis, diabetes, and back pain.

Treating OSA improves quality of life. A recent metaanalysis of 16 RCTs (total n = 1256) found that PAP enhanced overall vitality and physical domains of quality of life.[68]

Other sleep disorders

Obstructive sleep apnea is highly co-morbid with numerous other sleep disorders. For example, although chronic insomnia and OSA were once considered mutually exclusive, an increasing body of research has emerged demonstrating that they frequently co-exist.[69] Insomnia can interfere with PAP adherence[70] as well as treatment outcome from oral appliance therapy.[71] Cognitive behavioral treatment can be effective for patients experiencing co-morbid insomnia and poor PAP adherence.[72] OSA is also common in patients diagnosed with periodic limb movement disorder, and treatment via PAP can alleviate this.[73] Similarly, parasomnias may occur more frequently in patients with OSA, and can be improved with PAP.[74]

⚠ CAUTION

Presenting features of OSA can be subtle! Clinicians should have a high degree of suspicion and should ask specific sleep-related questions during assessment of all patients with high rates of known OSA co-morbidity: mood disorders, posttraumatic stress disorder, insomnia, and chronic pain. Many such patients do not present with typical signs of OSA such as obesity, loud snoring, or witnessed apneas. Instead, these patients may present with insomnia, soft snoring, increased fatigue, and somatic complaints, or higher levels of psychiatric distress. Older patients and postmenopausal women are also at much higher risk for occult OSA than premenopausal women and younger patients.

Conclusion

Obstructive sleep apnea is a chronic medical condition affecting multiple domains of physical, mental, and emotional function. Bidirectional relationships characterize many of the numerous consequences and co-morbidities associated with OSA. The often subtle presentations of OSA can make detection difficult; it is thus incumbent on healthcare professionals to be vigilant for screening for OSA and considering OSA as a contributing factor even in the absence of daytime sequelae. PAP therapy remains the gold standard treatment for OSA, and evidence suggests that PAP improves many of the medical consequences associated with OSA.

Disclaimer

The views expressed herein are those of the authors and do not reflect the official policy of the Department of the Army, Department of Defense, or the US Government.

References

1. Marshall NS, Wong KK, Liu PY, Cullen SR, Knuiman MW, Grunstein RR. Sleep apnea as an independent risk factor for all-cause mortality: the Busselton Health Study. *Sleep* 2008; **31**(8): 1079–85.

2. Punjabi NM, Caffo BS, Goodwin JL, et al. Sleep-disordered breathing and mortality: a prospective cohort study. PLoS Med 2009; **6**(8): e1000132. Epub Aug 18.

3. Marrone O, Lo Bue A, Salvaggio A, Dardanoni G, Insalaco G. Comorbidities and survival in obstructive sleep apnoea beyond the age of 50. *Eur J Clin Invest* 2012; doi: 10.1111/eci.12011. Epub Sep 24.

4. Campos-Rodriguez F, Peña-Griñan N, Reyes-Nuñez N, et al. Mortality in obstructive sleep apnea-hypopnea patients treated with positive airway pressure. *Chest* 2005; **128**(2): 624–33.

5. Campos-Rodriguez F, Martinez-Garcia MA, de la Cruz-Moron I, Almeida-Gonzalez C, Catalan-Serra P, Montserrat JM. Cardiovascular mortality in women with obstructive sleep apnea with or without continuous positive airway pressure treatment: a cohort study. *Ann Intern Med* 2012; **156**(2): 115–22.

6. Martínez-García MA, Campos-Rodríguez F, Catalán-Serra P, et al. Cardiovascular mortality in obstructive sleep apnea in the elderly: role of long-term continuous positive airway pressure treatment: a prospective observational study. *Am J Respir Crit Care Med* 2012; **186**(9): 909–16.

7. Wickwire EM. Behavioral management of sleep-disordered breathing. *Primary Psychiatry* 2009; **16**(2): 34–41.

8. Craig SE, Kohler M, Nicoll D, et al. Continuous positive airway pressure improves sleepiness but not calculated vascular risk in patients with minimally symptomatic obstructive sleep apnoea: the MOSAIC randomised controlled trial. *Thorax* 2012; **67**(12): 1090–6.

9. Wickwire EM, Lettieri CJ, Cairns AC, Collop NA. (2013). Maximizing PAP adherence in adults: a common-sense approach. *Chest* **144** (2), 680–693.

10. Brooks D, Horner RL, Kozar LF, Render-Teixeira CL, Phillipson EA. Obstructive sleep apnea as a cause of systemic hypertension. Evidence from a canine model. *J Clin Invest* 1997; **99**(1): 106–9.

11. Peppard PE, Young T, Palta M, Skatrud J. Prospective study of the association between sleep-disordered breathing and hypertension. *N Engl J Med* 2000; **342**(19): 1378–84.

12. Chobanian AV, Bakris GL, Black HR, et al. Seventh Report of the Joint National Committee on Prevention, Detection, Evaluation, and Treatment of High Blood Pressure. *Hypertension* 2003; **42**(6): 1206–52.

13. Becker HF, Jerrentrup A, Ploch T, et al. Effect of nasal continuous positive airway pressure treatment on blood pressure in patients with obstructive sleep apnea. *Circulation* 2003; **107**(1): 68–73.

14. Bazzano LA, Khan Z, Reynolds K, He J. Effect of nocturnal nasal continuous positive airway pressure on blood pressure in obstructive sleep apnea. *Hypertension* 2007; **50**(2): 417–23.

15. Davies CW, Crosby JH, Mullins RL, Barbour C, Davies RJ, Stradling JR. Case–control study of 24 hour ambulatory blood pressure in patients with obstructive sleep apnoea and normal matched control subjects. *Thorax* 2000; **55**(9): 736–40.

16. Gami AS, Howard DE, Olson EJ, Somers VK. Day-night pattern of sudden death in obstructive sleep apnea. *N Engl J Med* 2005; **352**(12): 1206–14.

17. Logan AG, Tkacova R, Perlikowski SM, et al. Refractory hypertension and sleep apnoea: effect of CPAP on blood pressure and baroreflex. *Eur Respir J* 2003; **21**(2): 241–7.

18. Collop N. The effect of obstructive sleep apnea on chronic medical disorders. *Cleve Clin J Med* 2007; **74**(1): 72–8. Erratum in: Cleve Clin J Med 2007; 74(8): 576.

19. Minai OA, Ricaurte B, Kaw R, et al. Frequency and impact of pulmonary hypertension in patients with obstructive sleep apnea syndrome. *Am J Cardiol* 2009; **104**(9): 1300–6.

20. Arias MA, García-Río F, Alonso-Fernández A, Martínez I, Villamor J. Pulmonary hypertension in obstructive sleep apnoea: effects of continuous positive airway pressure: a

randomized, controlled cross-over study. *Eur Heart J* 2006; **27**(9): 1106–13.

21. Mehra R, Benjamin EJ, Shahar E, et al., for the Sleep Heart Health Study. Association of nocturnal arrhythmias with sleep-disordered breathing: the Sleep Heart Health Study. *Am J Respir Crit Care Med* 2006; **173**(8): 910–16.

22. Monahan K, Storfer-Isser A, Mehra R, et al. Triggering of nocturnal arrhythmias by sleep-disordered breathing events. *J Am Coll Cardiol* 2009; **54**(19): 1797–804.

23. Hoyer FF, Lickfett LM, Mittmann-Braun E, et al. High prevalence of obstructive sleep apnea in patients with resistant paroxysmal atrial fibrillation after pulmonary vein isolation. *J Interv Card Electrophysiol* 2010; **29**(1): 37–41.

24. Patel D, Mohanty P, Di Biase L, et al. Safety and efficacy of pulmonary vein antral isolation in patients with obstructive sleep apnea: the impact of continuous positive airway pressure. *Circ Arrhythm Electrophysiol* 2010; **3**(5): 445–51.

25. Kanagala R, Murali NS, Friedman PA, et al. Obstructive sleep apnea and the recurrence of atrial fibrillation. *Circulation* 2003; **107**(20): 2589–94.

26. Ryan CM, Usui K, Floras JS, Bradley TD. Effect of continuous positive airway pressure on ventricular ectopy in heart failure patients with obstructive sleep apnoea. *Thorax* 2005; **60**(9): 781–5.

27. Kaneko Y, Floras JS, Usui K, et al. Cardiovascular effects of continuous positive airway pressure in patients with heart failure and obstructive sleep apnea. *N Engl J Med* 2003; **348**(13): 1233–41.

28. Khayat RN, Abraham WT, Patt B, Pu M, Jarjoura D. In-hospital treatment of obstructive sleep apnea during decompensation of heart failure. *Chest* 2009; **136**(4): 991–7.

29. Kourouklis SP, Vagiakis E, Paraskevaidis IA, et al. Effective sleep apnoea treatment improves cardiac function in patients with chronic heart failure. *Int J Cardiol* 2012; doi: pii: S0167-5273(12)01207-7.10.1016/j.ijcard.2012.09.101. Epub Oct 2.

30. Bradley TD, Floras JS. Obstructive sleep apnoea and its cardiovascular consequences. *Lancet* 2009 ; **373**(9657): 82–93.

31. Konecny T, Kuniyoshi FH, Orban M, et al. Under-diagnosis of sleep apnea in patients after acute myocardial infarction. *J Am Coll Cardiol* 2010; **56**(9): 742–3.

32. Shahar E, Whitney CW, Redline S, et al. Sleep-disordered breathing and cardiovascular disease: cross-sectional results of the Sleep Heart Health Study. *Am J Respir Crit Care Med* 2001; **163**(1): 19–25.

33. Punjabi NM, Caffo BS, Goodwin JL, et al. Sleep-disordered breathing and mortality: a prospective cohort study. *PLoS Med* 2009; **6**(8): e1000132.

34. Shah NA, Yaggi HK, Concato J, Mohsenin V. Obstructive sleep apnea as a risk factor for coronary events or cardiovascular death. *Sleep Breath* 2010; **14**(2): 131–6.

35. Marin JM, Carrizo SJ, Vicente E, Agusti AG. Long-term cardiovascular outcomes in men with obstructive sleep apnoea-hypopnoea with or without treatment with continuous positive airway pressure: an observational study. *Lancet* 2005; **365**(9464): 1046–53.

36. Yaggi HK, Concato J, Kernan WN, Lichtman JH, Brass LM, Mohsenin V. Obstructive sleep apnea as a risk factor for stroke and death. *N Engl J Med* 2005; **353**(19): 2034–41.

37. Redline S, Yenokyan G, Gottlieb DJ, et al. Obstructive sleep apnea-hypopnea and incident stroke: the Sleep Heart Health Study. *Am J Respir Crit Care Med* 2010; **182**(2): 269–77.

38. Cho JG, Witting PK, Verma M, et al. Tissue vibration induces carotid artery endothelial dysfunction: a mechanism linking snoring and carotid atherosclerosis? *Sleep* 2011; **34**(6): 751–7.

39. Dyken ME, Somers VK, Yamada T, Ren ZY, Zimmerman MB. Investigating the relationship between stroke and obstructive sleep apnea. *Stroke* 1996; **27**(3): 401–7.

40. Turkington PM, Allgar V, Bamford J, Wanklyn P, Elliott MW. Effect of upper airway obstruction in acute stroke on functional outcome at 6 months. *Thorax* 2004; **59**(5): 367–71.

41. Palombini L, Guilleminault C. Stroke and treatment with nasal CPAP. *Eur J Neurol* 2006; **13**(2): 198–200.

42. Ip MS, Lam B, Ng MM, Lam WK, Tsang KW, Lam KS. Obstructive sleep apnea is independently associated with insulin resistance. *Am J Respir Crit Care Med* 2002; **165**(5): 670–6.

43. Punjabi NM, Polotsky VY. Disorders of glucose metabolism in sleep apnea. *J Appl Physiol* 2005; **99**(5): 1998–2007.

44. Punjabi NM, Sorkin JD, Katzel LI, Goldberg AP, Schwartz AR, Smith PL. Sleep-disordered breathing and insulin resistance in middle-aged and overweight men. *Am J Respir Crit Care Med* 2002; **165**(5): 677–82.

45. Punjabi NM, Shahar E, Redline S, Gottlieb DJ, Givelber R, Resnick HE, Sleep Heart Health Study Investigators. Sleep-disordered breathing, glucose intolerance, and insulin resistance: the Sleep Heart Health Study. *Am J Epidemiol* 2004; **160**(6): 521–30.

46. Reichmuth KJ, Austin D, Skatrud JB, Young T. Association of sleep apnea and type II diabetes: a population-based study. *Am J Respir Crit Care Med* 2005; **172**(12): 1590–5.

47. Spiegel K, Knutson K, Leproult R, Tasali E, Van Cauter E. Sleep loss: a novel risk factor for insulin resistance and Type 2 diabetes. *J Appl Physiol* 2005; **99**(5): 2008–19.

48. Newman AB, Foster G, Givelber R, Nieto FJ, Redline S, Young T. Progression and regression of sleep-disordered breathing with changes in weight: the Sleep Heart Health Study. *Arch Intern Med* 2005; **165**(20): 2408–13.

49. Yang D, Liu Z, Yang H, Luo Q. Effects of continuous positive airway pressure on glycemic control and insulin resistance in patients with obstructive sleep apnea: a meta-analysis. *Sleep Breath* 2013; **17**(1): 33–8.

50. Quan SF, Chan CS, Dement WC, et al. The association between obstructive sleep apnea and neurocognitive performance – the Apnea Positive Pressure Long-term Efficacy Study (APPLES). *Sleep* 2011; **34**(3): 303–14B.

51. Beebe DW, Groesz L, Wells C, Nichols A, McGee K. The neuropsychological effects of obstructive sleep apnea: a meta-analysis of norm-referenced and case-controlled data. *Sleep* 2003; **26**(3): 298–307.

52. Mazza S, Pépin JL, Naëgelé B, Plante J, Deschaux C, Lévy P. Most obstructive sleep apnoea patients exhibit vigilance and attention deficits on an extended battery of tests. *Eur Respir J* 2005; **25**(1): 75–80.

53. Naëgelé B, Launois SH, Mazza S, Feuerstein C, Pépin JL, Lévy P. Which memory processes are affected in patients with obstructive sleep apnea? An evaluation of 3 types of memory. *Sleep* 2006; **29**(4): 533–44.

54. Ayalon L, Ancoli-Israel S, Aka AA, McKenna BS, Drummond SP. Relationship between obstructive sleep apnea severity and brain activation during a sustained attention task. *Sleep* 2009; **32**(3): 373–81.

55. Archbold KH, Borghesani PR, Mahurin RK, Kapur VK, Landis CA. Neural activation patterns during working memory tasks and OSA disease severity: preliminary findings. *J Clin Sleep Med* 2009; **5**(1): 21–7.

56. Salorio CF, White DA, Piccirillo J, Duntley SP, Uhles ML. Learning, memory, and executive control in individuals with obstructive sleep apnea syndrome. *J Clin Exp Neuropsychol* 2002; **24**(1): 93–100.

57. Aloia MS, Arnedt JT, Davis JD, Riggs RL, Byrd D. Neuropsychological sequelae of obstructive sleep apnea-hypopnea syndrome: a critical review. *J Int Neuropsychol Soc* 2004; **10**(5): 772–85.

58. Zimmerman ME, Arnedt JT, Stanchina M, Millman RP, Aloia MS. Normalization of memory performance and positive airway pressure adherence in memory-impaired patients with obstructive sleep apnea. *Chest* 2006; **130**(6): 1772–8.

59. Young T, Blustein J, Finn L, Palta M. Sleep-disordered breathing and motor vehicle accidents in a population-based sample of employed adults. *Sleep* 1997; **20**(8): 608–13.

60. Tregear S, Reston J, Schoelles K, Phillips B. Continuous positive airway pressure reduces risk of motor vehicle crash among drivers with obstructive sleep apnea: systematic review and meta-analysis. *Sleep* 2010; **33**(10): 1373–80.

61. Saunamäki T, Jehkonen M. Depression and anxiety in obstructive sleep apnea syndrome: a review. *Acta Neurol Scand* 2007; **116**(5): 277–88.

62. Sharafkhaneh A, Giray N, Richardson P, Young T, Hirshkowitz M. Association of psychiatric disorders and sleep apnea in a large cohort. *Sleep* 2005; **28**(11): 1405–11.

63. Alam A, Chengappa KN, Ghinassi F. Screening for obstructive sleep apnea among individuals with severe mental illness at a primary care clinic. *Gen Hosp Psychiatry* 2012; **34**(6): 660–4.

64. Ohayon MM. The effects of breathing-related sleep disorders on mood disturbances in the general population. *J Clin Psychiatry* 2003; **64**(10): 1195–200; quiz, 1274–6.

65. Haba-Rubio J. Psychiatric aspects of organic sleep disorders. *Dialogues Clin Neurosci* 2005; **7**(4): 335–46.

66. Cross RL, Kumar R, Macey PM, et al. Neural alterations and depressive symptoms in obstructive sleep apnea patients. *Sleep* 2008; **31**(8): 1103–9.

67. Finn L, Young T, Palta M, Fryback DG. Sleep-disordered breathing and self-reported general health status in the Wisconsin Sleep Cohort Study. *Sleep* 1998; **21**(7): 701–6.

68. Jing J, Huang T, Cui W, Shen H. Effect on quality of life of continuous positive airway pressure in patients with obstructive sleep apnea syndrome: a meta-analysis. *Lung* 2008; **186**(3): 131–44.

69. Wickwire EM, Collop NA. Insomnia and sleep-related breathing disorders. *Chest* 2010; **137**(6): 1449–63.

70. Wickwire EM, Smith MT, Birnbaum S, Collop NA. Sleep maintenance insomnia complaints predict poor CPAP adherence: a clinical case series. *Sleep Med* 2010; **11**(8): 772–6.

71. Machado MA, de Carvalho LB, Juliano ML, Taga M, do Prado LB, do Prado GF. Clinical co-morbidities in obstructive sleep apnea syndrome treated with mandibular repositioning appliance. *Respir Med* 2006; **100**(6): 988–95.

72. Wickwire EM, Schumacher JA, Richert AC, Baran AS, Roffwarg HP. Combined insomnia and poor CPAP compliance: a case study and discussion. *Clin Case Stud* 2008; **7**(4): 267–86.

73. Baran AS, Richert AC, Douglass AB, May W, Ansarin K. Change in periodic limb movement index during treatment of obstructive sleep apnea with continuous positive airway pressure. *Sleep* 2003; **26**(6): 717–20.

74. Guilleminault C, Hagen CC, Khaja AM. Catathrenia: parasomnia or uncommon feature of sleep disordered breathing? *Sleep* 2008; **31**(1): 132–9.

9

Non-Pharmacological Treatments of Insomnia and Circadian Rhythm Disorder: Special Focus on Neurology Patients

Mary Rose, PsyD, CBSM

Department of Medicine, Pulmonary, Critical Care and Sleep Medicine, Baylor College of Medicine, USA

Introduction

Of all the sleep disorders, insomnia is the most ubiquitous. A general consensus developed from population-based studies suggests that about 30% of adult sampled report insomnia.[1] When only those with daytime impairment or distress consequent to insomnia were considered, the National Institutes of Health State of the Science Conference found an approximately 10% prevalence of insomnia.[2] Arguments for the cost and health benefits of treating insomnia are well established. Those with insomnia report overall impaired quality of life,[3] increased utilization of medical services,[4] and greater absenteeism from work.[5]

Research on insomnia in those with neurological problems is relatively limited, but insomnia is known to be a common complaint in many types of neurological disorders, including epilepsy, movement disorders, and neurodegenerative conditions. Sleep is sensitive to both psychosocial challenge and medical compromise. Neurological illnesses may compromise mood, memory, and cognitive processing, adding an additional barrier to both achieving an adequate quality of sleep and frustration tolerance for poor sleep and the associated fatigue.

As with insomnia, circadian rhythm sleep disorders (CRSD) are highly receptive to non-pharmacological treatment, and this has been gaining some recent investigative progress with regard to neurological disorders. Circadian disorders are often misdiagnosed as insomnia. Many clinicians are not as familiar with the available options (both behavioral and pharmacological) for the treatment of CRSD. In neurological patients, circadian rhythm disorders may play a role in magnifying some ancillary aspects of their primary disorder or sleep complaint such as restless legs syndrome (RLS) which in turn magnify insomnia symptoms.

The major focus of this chapter is identification of insomnia and review of the use of non-pharmacological therapies to facilitate the treatment of insomnia, particularly in those with co-morbid neurological disorders. Though less of a focus, circadian rhythm disorders will also be reviewed, as they are common, manifest as difficulty with sleep timing, and are amenable to cognitive behavioral interventions.

Some of the most common neurological illnesses in which insomnia and circadian rhythm disorders are problematic include multiple sclerosis (MS), Alzheimer's disease (AD), and Parkinson's disease (PD). Though sleep is sensitive to migraines, seizures, and other neurological illnesses, MS, AD, and PD appear to be commonly associated with insomnia and circadian disruption; frequently these patients are referred to sleep centers. In fact, sleep disruption is of great enough clinical interest to

Sleep Medicine in Neurology, First Edition. Edited by Douglas B. Kirsch.
© 2014 John Wiley & Sons, Ltd. Published 2014 by John Wiley & Sons, Ltd.

patients with these disorders and the practitioners who care for them that the National Sleep Foundation has featured information for each of these neurological disorders on their web page under *Sleep Topics*.

Insomnia

Diagnostic definitions of insomnia

The *International Classification of Sleep Disorders* (ICSD-2)[6] differentiates multiple diagnostic categories of insomnia (Box 9.1). Most of these are consistent with the *International Classification of Diseases* (ICD)-9 subcategories of insomnia. In the ICD-9 the most commonly used global diagnostic category for insomnia is *Persistent Disorder of Initiating or Maintaining Sleep*. This is described as hyposomnia, insomnia, or sleeplessness associated with anxiety, conditioned arousal, depression, psychosis, idiopathic insomnia, paradoxical insomnia, primary insomnia, or psychophysiological insomnia. Requirements for insomnia include a complaint of difficulty getting or staying asleep or having non-restorative sleep. A sleep efficiency of less than 85% (the total percent of time the patient sleeps during the night) is one strategy for determining the combination of sleep onset latency and wake after sleep onset. Symptoms must be present for three or more nights per week and be associated with a ≥30 min sleep onset latency (SOL) or wake after sleep onset (WASO). The duration of insomnia should be greater than 6 months. The effects of insomnia should be distressing and an impediment socially, emotionally, and/or occupationally. This latter criterion is critical because it is often neglected in clinical interview. As with most psychological diagnosis, distress and impairment are essential consequences of the disorder.

Particularly in the neurological patient, sorting out the causes of a sleep disturbance requires both time and detective work. To identify the source of insomnia, the clinician should first decipher if symptoms are *primary* or *secondary* (Box 9.2). The ICD-9 classification carries a broad code for *Persistent Disorder of Initiating or Maintaining Sleep*, which is inclusive of a multitude of possible causes for insomnia, including primary, psychophysiological, organic, idiopathic, with obstructive sleep apnea (OSA), medication induced, alcohol induced, drug induced, mental disorders, etc. One advantage to this is that it acknowledges that insomnia, with its dual role as both a disease and a symptom, is often mediated by a rich dynamic of biobehavioral causes. However, it is essential to ensure that there is no other disorder which has not yet been identified or treated which is the primary factor driving the insomnia. Presence of another disorder does not preclude psychophysiological insomnia, but may complicate progress with treatment if the other disorders are not also adeptly addressed.

Assignment of a specific diagnosis of insomnia (for example, primary *psychophysiological insomnia* which assumes a mind–body interaction, but that a primary anxiety disorder or medical cause is not the central cause) is often misleading as multiple factors are typically at play, not only in the neurology

---

Box 9.1 ICSD-2 types

Adjustment insomnia
Psychophysiological insomnia
Paradoxical insomnia
Idiopathic insomnia
Insomnia due to a mental disorder
Inadequate sleep hygiene
Behavioral insomnia of childhood
Insomnia due to a drug or substance
Insomnia due to a medical disorder
Insomnia not due to substance or known
    physiological condition
Physiological (organic) insomnia, unspecified

Box 9.2 Secondary insomnia: common psychological and medical causes

Psychological	Medical
Anxiety: generalized, panic, obsessive compulsive disorder	Obstructive sleep apnea
Depression	Periodic limb movement disorder
Alcohol abuse	Thyroid disease
Bipolar	Multiple sclerosis
	Parkinson's disease
	Dementia
	Headache disorder

patient but in many patients seen in a primary care setting. One beneficial aspect of a primary and secondary classification is that it may guide the clinician with priority setting how specific aspects of sleep disturbance might be addressed. Attempting to classify insomnia as insomnia *specifically* due to a medical cause or medication is often also a risky assumption, unless the patient was clearly without complaint of insomnia until an acute exacerbation or treatment with known insomnia protagonists such as solumedrol.

An insomnia assessment should include not only evaluation of the factors involved in the sleep disturbance, but the patient's readiness for change, capacity for insight-oriented management of symptoms, and tolerance for change and frustration. Each of these is critical to successfully identifying and reaching goals.

☆ TIPS AND TRICKS

Previsit questionnaires

A previsit questionnaire will not only save time during a clinical interview but may facilitate disclosure of common contributors to insomnia that are not easily divulged during interview. These may include mood symptoms such as unhappiness, anxiety, anhedonia, low sex drive, difficulty turning mind off at night, weight changes, lack of interest in usual things. Additional possible contributors to insomnia include a snoring partner, noise in the home, health problems, pain.

In addition to the standard questions for insomnia to differentiate difficulty initiating and maintaining sleep from early morning wakes, general sleep hygiene questions, the influence of pain, meds and medical conditions on insomnia, the practitioner may better illuminate insomnia by expanding their query to include additional aspects of the environment, cognitions surrounding sleep and tapping into patient awareness of what affects sleep (Box 9.3).

Specific identification and weighing of the degree to which medical conditions, other sleep disorders, psychological adjustment, stressors (e.g. stress about disease progression, physical handicap, social stigma, existential crisis), and pain contribute

---

Box 9.3 Insomnia questions

Do any of your bed partners, pets or human, disrupt your sleep?

Do you keep a light and/or a TV on during the night?

Do you have difficulty with worry at night (about things that might happen)?

Do you have difficulty turning your mind off at night?

Do you ruminate at night (think about things that have happened)?

Do you fear the bedroom/bedtime or sleep?

---

to a sleep disturbance is a challenge for the provider and patient. Typically, causes of insomnia are multifaceted, synergistic, and rarely attributable to a single etiology. Thus, the patient's complaint of insomnia requires a careful review of history and symptoms, and will determine the course of treatment. Though the course often involves the main standard of care techniques, how they are implemented may vary.

Timing of insomnia episodes during the night is diagnostically important. Sleep-onset difficulty is often significantly related to diurnal anxiety, hyperarousal, and poor sleep habits. Middle-of-sleep awakenings may be related to co-morbid medical problems such as nocturnal leg cramps, nocturia, periodic limb movement, sleep-disordered breathing, pain, hot flashes, and medication, though habits and mood symptoms cannot be eliminated. Early morning spontaneous waking is a hallmark symptom of depression, but may also be an indication of circadian shift or simply environmental factors such as noise. Early morning waking may also flag possible rapid eye movement (REM)-related obstructive sleep apnea.

For the neurological patient, a critical symptom that is often intermeshed with the sleep complaint is fatigue. For some neurological disorders such as MS, presence of fatigue (as measured by the Fatigue Descriptive Scale) has been found to be strongly correlated with presence of both insomnia and circadian rhythm disorders.[7] Multiple other factors such as a change in the progression of illness, visibility of symptoms (ex: spasticity) and/or medication transitions may all be at play in the worsening of emotional, physical, and cognitive fatigue. This is turn magnifies sleep disturbance as the patient copes with these new stressors. Patients in warm climates with MS may also experience Uhthoff's related fatigue and worsening of symptoms which may in turn magnify sleep complaints.

Insomnia and mood disturbance in the general population

Depression, anxiety, and sleep disturbance are often interwoven. In a major population study, 14,915 subjects were sampled from the general population in the United Kingdom, Germany, Italy, and Portugal, and extensive interviews were conducted to assess mental health and sleep parameters.[8] Investigators found that 28% of those with insomnia had a concurrent diagnosis of a mental disorder, and 25.6% had history of a psychiatric disorder. Presence of severe insomnia, diagnosis of primary insomnia, insomnia related to a medical condition, and insomnia that lasted more than 1 year predicted a psychiatric history in this study. Insomnia is a significant predictor of depression. In most cases where a mood disorder was present, insomnia appeared prior to (>40%) or concurrently with (>22%) mood disorder symptoms. This finding suggests that the early physiological changes of depression may manifest in architectural changes to sleep.[8]

In another study, 17–50% of subjects with insomnia that had lasted 2 weeks or longer developed a major depressive episode at the time of later interview.[9] In a review of more than 250 journal articles, Tsuno's dramatic finding that the co-morbidity of insomnia with depression occurred in about 90% of patients with depression[10] provides further evidence that impaired sleep drive is a hallmark of mood disturbance. These studies suggest that for those at risk of depression, insomnia is not only often a prequel to depression but may be a risk factor for those undergoing stressful life events.

Findings on depression and insomnia fit well into a diathesis-stress model of insomnia. This model suggests that diathesis (individual factors which may function as vulnerabilities) interact with a stressful event to provoke expression of the sleep disturbance. This will be discussed later with regard to Spielman's three-factor model of insomnia. In those with neurological problems, stress may worsen the symptoms and in turn sleep quality and quantity.

Risk factors such as anxious personality, poor coping, lack of social support, and depression will most certainly make one more vulnerable to insomnia. Fragile or light sleep, (that which is susceptible to noise, light, temperature variations, movement of a bed partner, etc.) may magnify these problems in an already hypervigilant patient.

Polysomnography and physiological markers and insomnia

Over the past decade, we have learned considerably more about the pathophysiology of insomnia. Polysomnography suggests that the sleep of those with primary insomnia differs from that of good sleepers in several ways. Feige et al. showed overall impairment of sleep architecture, including increased arousal during REM sleep.[11] In addition to electrical differences in brain activity, patients with primary insomnia tend to be hypermetabolic, running at a persistently slightly higher metabolic rate than age-matched controls.[12] This finding is of interest with regard to developing a treatment plan targeting features of insomnia such as inability to "turn off" and wind down. It is possible that the hypermetabolic status of the insomnia patient is reflective of the general difficulty these patients have with disconnecting themselves physically and mentally to allow relaxation and the associated sleep that ensues.

Sleepiness or fatigue?

Typically, fatigue is defined as a mental and/or physical weariness, while sleepiness is defined as a propensity to fall asleep and difficulty maintaining wakefulness. Sleep quality and daytime sleepiness have been found to be good predictors of fatigue in multiple regression analysis.[13] However, clinically, insomnia tends to be routinely associated with fatigue and is infrequently associated with sleepiness to the same degree. Fatigue is a well-known secondary effect of many neurological conditions including MS and PD. The reader is cautioned to clarify these symptoms with patients as much as possible; even the literature on sleep and fatigue often blends them interchangeably.

Pharmacological management of insomnia: the basics

Most sleep experts do not routinely recommend long-term benzodiazepine (BZD) hypnotics or non-BZD hypnotics for insomnia. Research by Morin et al. suggests that a combined approach to medication and cognitive behavioral therapy for insomnia (CBT-I) was *initially* beneficial in alleviating symptoms. However, subjects who continued maintenance CBT-I after initial treatment for insomnia and tapered their medication during extended therapy achieved the best outcome results. These patients also obtained better long-term outcomes compared to those who continued using medication, even intermittently.[14] The reader interested in an extensive review of the use of BZD and non-BZD hypnotics in the treatment of insomnia is referred to Thase[15] and Perlis et al.[16]

One of the fundamental barriers to progress in insomnia, as with anxiety disorders, is the patient's belief that they are not in control over their emotions, and that only outside forces (e.g. medication and the influence of others) can manage the symptoms. Lack of insight regarding how one's thoughts and behaviors influence insomnia (as well as general anxiety) is disabling to progress. BZD and non-BZD hypnotics have not been found to be effective overall for long-term treatment of insomnia,[17] possibly due to the fact that intense dysfunctional thoughts about sleep (which often brood during waking hours) and maladaptive associations with sleep and the bedroom are so intensely conditioned that they are resistant to pharmacological eradication.

Mood disturbance and insomnia in neurological patients

The most prevalent psychological co-morbities with insomnia include anxiety and depression. The prominence of mood disturbance in some neurological conditions is an important consideration as it affects not only how the sleep disturbance is expressed but how it may affect the direction of treatment.

Several studies have suggested that MS is associated with mood disturbance. Self-reported rates vary, but have been found to be about 57% for depression,[18,19] and 63% for anxiety.[18] Studies suggest a 34–46% rate of depressive disorder[20,21] and a 44% prevalence of anxiety symptoms 44%.[21] However, Chahraoui et al. also found alexithymia (deficiency in understanding, processing, or describing emotions) to be prominent in MS patients.[21] More variability with sleep and mood may exist in benign and relapsing remitting forms versus primary progressive

courses of the disease. Some studies suggest that overall sleep quality in MS patients is associated with pain, greater disease severity, and poorer mental and physical quality of life.[22]

Insomnia is likewise common in patients with PD,[23] though there are mixed data on the severity of PD over time with the course of insomnia.[24] PD patients appear to have greater problems with frequent nocturnal awakenings than with sleep onset.[25] Factor et al. did not find statistically significant differences between patients with PD and healthy elderly controls with regard to difficulty initiating sleep (67% versus 54%) though sleep fragmentation was common in patients with PD (89% versus 74%), marked by more frequent nocturnal awakenings than in controls (2–5 awakenings in PD patients versus 1–3 per night for controls).[23]

Additional causes of insomnia in neurological diseases

Patients with neurological conditions may experience excessive daytime sleepiness or insomnia for a variety of reasons. Primary causes of sleep-wake disorders in many neurologically compromised patients include medication and/or disease processes (including pain). During treatment, MS patients often experience episodic insomnia, particularly with use of intravenous (IV) steroids during treatment for symptomatic flare-ups. Disease-modifying medications may also have the side-effects of insomnia. Small samples suggest that 25–54% of MS patients experience insomnia.[22] Nocturnal leg cramps and restless legs syndrome may also add to reports of insomnia, though the effect of these are not well studied in this population.

Dopaminergic drugs used for RLS, PD, and other movement disorders may also cause the side-effect of excessive daytime sleepiness. Stocchi et al. found that when levodopa/carbidopa was administered at bedtime, sleep quality was improved substantially.[26] For an excellent review of insomnia in patients with neurodegenerative conditions, the reader is referred to Dauvilliers.[27]

Non-pharmacological treatment of insomnia

The American Academy of Sleep Medicine has indicated that stimulus control therapy (SCT), cognitive behavioral therapy, and relaxation training be considered standard of care for insomnia treatment.

Sleep restriction, multicomponent therapy (without cognitive therapy), paradoxical intention, and biofeedback were deemed guidelines. The report states that the use of imagery training and sleep hygiene have not provided enough evidence to support their use as single therapies.[28] A later update of these metaanalyses suggests that of the five, SCT and cognitive behavioral therapy have the most significant benefit on the treatment of insomnia.[29]

Sleep hygiene

It is critical at this juncture to emphasize that cognitive behavioral therapy (CBT) generally includes a combination of modalities. Patient and clinician alike often confuse sleep hygiene with CBT. The danger in confusing these treatments is that many providers administer sleep hygiene handouts identifying them as CBT-I. Sleep hygiene is composed of simple rules for improving sleep behaviorally, though they do incorporate some elements of stimulus control instruction (Box 9.4). However, sleep hygiene recommendations alone

---

Box 9.4 Common sleep hygiene recommendations

1. Reduce or eliminate caffeine after noon. Avoid alcohol and nicotine close to bedtime.
2. Avoid TV or other arousing activities in the bedroom.
3. Avoid having disruptive pets in bed.
4. Keep a regular routine on weekdays and weekends.
5. Establish a regular, relaxing bedtime routine.
6. Keep the bedroom dark, quiet, comfortable, and cool.
7. Use your bedroom only for sleep and sex.
8. Exercise regularly; finish a few hours before bedtime.
9. Avoid naps.
10. Go to bed only when sleepy.
11. Designate a time to write down problems and solutions earlier in the day, not close to bedtime.
12. After about 20 minutes of not being able to get to sleep, go to another room to read until sleepy.

---

are not deemed effective for the treatment of chronic insomnia.

Sleep hygiene handouts should be carefully reviewed with patients before being given out to identify both which behaviors are most beneficial to target for *that* patient and which behaviors the patient is ready to change.

Sleep restriction/sleep compression

An essential part of the behavioral treatment of insomnia is sleep restriction or sleep compression. Sleep restriction serves the role of restricting time in bed to only sleep. The clinician determines the total sleep time and then modifies the sleep schedule to include only the time that the patient reports sleeping. Sleep compression, in which the clinician draws the time in bed in around the total hours of sleep, is often used in lieu of sleep restriction. This is particularly important when modifying the schedule of a patient who is highly anxious or who otherwise may be too resistant to the sleep restriction to participate in the scheduled sleep time. Patients will often protest that they want to *rest* in bed in the absence of sleep. This provides the opportunity for the clinician to remind the patient of the concepts behind the SCT intervention.

★ TIPS AND TRICKS

Introducing sleep restriction

Link the rationale to SCT by reminding the patient that if they are not sleeping then remaining in bed serves only to:

1. strengthen the association between wake and the bedroom
2. further intensify frustration and aggravation about not sleeping.

Stimulus control therapy

The first line of treatment for chronic insomnia is stimulus control therapy (SCT). SCT postulates that it is the paired association between the sleep environment (bedroom) and the learned arousal that perpetuates hyperarousal and insomnia. Detaching the association by removing oneself from the environment but not engaging in sleep outside the bedroom is the key feature to stimulus control therapy. The strategies discussed herein are identical to those used with otherwise healthy insomnia

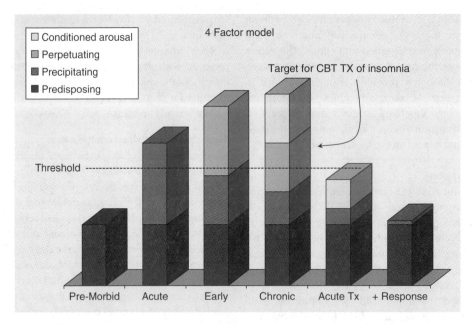

Figure 9.1 Spielman model modified to include premorbid, acute treatment and response. From Perlis M, Jungquist C, Smith M, Posner D. *Cognitive Behavioral Treatment of Insomnia*, 2005. Reproduced with permission of Springer Science and Business Media.

patients, with some minor modifications specific to those with neurological patients.

Bootzin first published his treatment of SCT in 1972.[30] STC proposes that reconditioning maladaptive associations with the sleep environment is an essential feature of insomnia. A major premise for SCT is that remaining in bed while not sleeping sets up a classical conditioning scenario. Thus, the patient associates the state of wakefulness with the bed and bedroom, which in turn reinforces inability to sleep.

Spielman's three-factor model of insomnia is a widely accepted, largely temporally based conceptualization of insomnia (Figure 9.1). This model postulates that insomnia is influenced by predisposing, precipitating, and perpetuating factors.[31] It proposes the mechanism through which insomnia transitions from an acute to a chronic condition through thoughts and behaviors. Thus, an individual is often vulnerable to insomnia consequent upon trait characteristics. An episode of insomnia is triggered by a precipitating factor such as a significant life event, and perpetuated consequent to dysfunctional behavioral and cognitive patterns that are maladaptive.

Cognitive behavioral therapy for insomnia

Cognitive behavioral therapy targeted specifically at insomnia (CBT-I) has been shown to be highly effective in modifying dysfunctional cognitions related to sleep. Research on insomnia with co-morbid depression suggests that CBT-I enhanced outcome on depression measures in those with major depression disorder.[32] Numerous studies have indicated that CBT-I is a highly effective treatment compared with sleep hygiene alone.[33] The cognitive behavioral model of insomnia developed by Morin identifies two mechanisms of CBT specifically for insomnia: the reduction of dysfunctional beliefs about sleep and maladaptive sleep behaviors. SCT targets the maladaptive associations formed under the classical conditioning scenario of paired association between the bedroom environment and the arousal. Cognitive therapy moves this forward to target maladaptive associations with sleep itself for cognitive modification.

The most essential cognitive features of insomnia that require attention include worry (focus on potential bad experiences for the future) and ruminations (focus on bad experiences from the past), misperceptions about sleep, monitoring threat, and dysfunctional beliefs about sleep. Worry and rumination have been shown to benefit from both the conditions of a structured proactive problem solving, or in completion of a worry questionnaire.[34] This finding suggests, to at least some degree, that diurnal avoidance may be a component of perpetuating insomnia. Initially, many patients deny diurnal anxiety and/or that anxiety may be contributing to insomnia, likely due to fear that their symptoms will be dismissed as secondary.

Many patients are guarded about their anxious thoughts and habits. Comprehensive interview, involvement of family, and building rapport are critical to uncovering underlying symptoms. Certainly, for patients vulnerable to mood disturbance, insomnia is a risk factor when they are faced with the consequences of neuropsychiatric change, social upheaval, physical changes, loss of income, and job security.

Sometimes the clinician must carefully review the history of symptoms, and when the history is nebulous, cue the patient with questions such as "so you weren't sleeping well 5 years ago, tell me about what was happening and how you were sleeping 6 years ago."

Often patients are able to recognize that a likely reason for worry and ruminations emerging once they are in bed or nearing the bedroom is due to lack of being otherwise refocused or distracted with the events of the day. As is the nature of avoidance, pending concerns or seemingly insurmountable barriers loom unaddressed and strike the patient when they are most vulnerable. This, magnified with the paired association between the bedroom and wake, becomes a powerful stimulant. During the daytime the patient may think about sleep catastrophically and fear the bedroom. Often, insomnia patients cite counterproductive strategies to obtain sleep. One of the most common is trying to "force sleep." The desperation and overempowerment of the insomnia that patients give sleep is often magnified by other strategies such as "begging and praying to God that I will sleep." These strategies typically provide little comfort and fail because they remove control from the patient. They additionally do not engage the patient in a proactive strategy for either correction of dysfunctional beliefs or management of hyperarousal. In his patient-centered book on Insomnia, Espie talks about "automaticity" of sleep.[35] Automaticity is a skill that Espie notes good sleepers have in common. Sleep for those without

complaint is experienced much like any other drive, and they follow it without much thought or difficulty. In the insomnia patient, however, the drive of sleep has disconnected from the automaticity, leaving the person with a malfunctioning off switch.

Treatment plan

A detailed history is critical before an optimal treatment plan for insomnia can be developed. One of the most essential features of non-pharmacological treatment of insomnia is that it requires patient understanding of the concepts of how insomnia may be influenced by predisposing, precipitating, and perpetuating factors. In addition to identifying the pattern of symptoms and keeping sleep journals and records of ruminative thoughts proactively, the patient must be ready to change habits and thoughts. See Figure 9.2 for a decision tree on differential diagnosis and treatment planning.

Knowing as much as possible about the factors influencing the patient's sleep, as well as what the patient has tried in the past to alleviate symptoms, is essential in building rapport and designing a proper individualized treatment plan. Unlike most medical and psychiatric disorders, those with insomnia have often been faced with varying degrees of partial treatment, ineffective online self-treatment, misleading reading materials, and a plethora of medications. These problems forge a guarded and challenging patient. This is largely because standard of care for most common psychiatric and medical diseases is not only well established, but access to providers who routinely implement treatment is not as challenging as it is with insomnia. For the neurological patient with insomnia, there is the added treatment challenge of a larger repertoire of medications than is typical in the general population, and with often a greater cache of physical obstacles and health unknowns.

Cognitive behavioral therapy for insomnia (multicomponent) ideally involves 6–8 weekly sessions. In practicality, many patients or practices may be unable to conduct weekly sessions and opt for bimonthly ones. The risk of foregoing weekly sessions is that patients may be vulnerable to dropout if they lose sight of progress and goals, or if they encounter an obstacle they feel unable to overcome. At each visit, progress should be reviewed. Treatment of insomnia should involve the keeping of sleep journals so that patients can track sleep patterns and progress over time. Goals also should

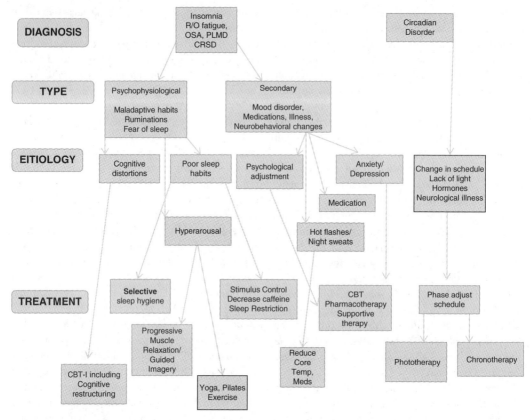

Figure 9.2 Insomnia Treatment Decision Tree.

be reevaluated frequently to reaffirm progress and to reappraise current status with sleep. This ensures that the patient does not lose sight of their ability to enact change (even small incremental ones).

Resistance to change may have complicated reasons. Even unhealthy habits may become familiar and incorporated into one's identity. Goals should be regularly revisited and resistance to making change should be *gently* explored. Patients with secondary gain to insomnia (an excuse to miss social obligations, being removed from the bedroom and a partner with whom there is conflict, etc.) are likely to resist progress.

Additional behavioral therapies

Guided imagery has not, in metaanalysis, been found to be effective in treatment of insomnia.[36]

However, we have found it effective for patients clinically in some cases. A likely mechanism of guided imagery is not only relaxation but redirecting dysfunctional and ruminative thoughts to a more productive line of focus. Patients with limited abstraction skills and poor visualization are not ideal candidates. Progressive muscle relaxation has been found in metaanalysis to be supported as a guideline.[37] It is recommended that once guided imagery and progressive muscle relaxation are explained, patients be given the option of which they feel would be most beneficial. One of the added benefits of this is that it requires some introspection and challenge to the patient, in that they must actively engage and participate in the treatment decision making as well as challenging themselves to engage in new therapies.

Paradoxical intention and biofeedback were judged to be guidelines by the AASM,[37] and are often used in multicomponent behavioral therapy. Paradoxical intention involves having the patient deliberately face the feared behavior by deliberately engaging in wake and actively avoiding sleep. Sleep restriction alone has not been indicated as an effective treatment, though it may be a powerful tool used as part of a multicomponent treatment.[37] Though not readily used at the time of the 1999 practice parameter paper on insomnia, sleep compression, in which the patient's time in bed is slowly closed in around the time of sleep, is routinely used as part of a multicomponent treatment.

> ✋ CAUTION
>
> Sleep restriction below 5 hours of total sleep time is not recommended.

Largely, the basic principles of non-pharmacological treatment of insomnia that are used with otherwise healthy patients should be applied to those who are medically compromised as well. Though there may be mitigating factors such as pain, medication, and the disease process itself, once these are addressed as well as possible, the patient, regardless of complication level, is still likely to benefit from implementing the basic principles of non-pharmacological treatment.

As previously noted, alexithymia appears to be more prevalent in those with MS than in the general population. This would present even greater difficulty in the patient's identification of feelings and sensations such as worry or dysphoria. Alexithymia may even compromise the ability to discriminate feelings of fatigue versus sleepiness. Some otherwise healthy insomnia patients struggle with identification of physical cues for sleepiness and must essentially be guided to be more observant to these cues. In patients who are compromised with regard to equilibrium, vigilance, and mood, this task becomes a challenge.

Circadian rhythm disorder

Diagnostic definitions of circadian rhythm disorder

There are several types of circadian rhythm sleep disorders (CRSD) identified by the ICSD-2. The most common include delayed sleep phase type, advanced sleep phase type, shift work type, irregular sleep-wake type, free-running type, and jet-lag type.

The clinician is most likely to see the first three of these disorders. The ICSD-2 indicates that "The essential feature of CRSDs is a persistent or recurrent pattern of sleep disturbance due primarily to alterations in the circadian timekeeping system or a misalignment between the endogenous circadian rhythm and exogenous factors that affect the timing or duration of sleep."[6]

Circadian disorders are present when the patient has a substantial delay or advance in the ideal timing of sleep. As with insomnia, diagnosis must involve impairment to occupational or social life. Delayed phase syndrome is most prominent in adolescence, while advanced phase is more common in older adults.

> ✋ CAUTION
>
> Circadian rhythm disorder (CRD) is often misdiagnosed as insomnia. The age of the patient and the total sleep time will alert the clinician that CRD may be the underlying problem.

Behavioral and pharmacological treatment of circadian rhythm disorders

Patients most often present with delayed phase sleep (falling asleep later than desired). This is most common in adolescents, and in fact is a natural phase shift.[38] Less often, patients present with a phase advance which is typically most distressing because of the early morning waking. As with insomnia, use of journals and sometimes actigraphy is highly useful in tracking the patient's sleep.

Chronotherapy, by which the patient is incrementally delayed in their sleep time over a period of several days to weeks and transitioned to their desired sleep time, is a standard of care.[39] This treatment may be impractical in working adults, unless performed during a vacation period. The reader is reminded that forcing wake is easier than forcing sleep when readjusting a schedule. Sleep drive will generally intensify if the patient is woken earlier and not allowed to nap.

Phototherapy is used to facilitate the advanced or delayed schedule. In delayed sleep phase syndrome, bright light administered in the early morning upon waking has been shown to facilitate the shift to an earlier sleep time (phase advance).[40] Often bright light therapy (blue light wavelength) with a luminance of 2500 lux is recommended.[41] Clinically, it is sometimes more practical to encourage routine daylight exposure during intended waking hours for those with regular daytime schedules. However, for patients with shift work sleep disorder, light boxes and bright light exposure during work are optimal. Careful blocking of light surrounding time of intended sleep (use of blue blocker sunglasses on the way home and blackout shades on bedroom windows) is also critical.

Behaviorally, patients need to regularize their schedule and to avoid the prioritizing of other activities (the tendency for which is strong in those working long nightshift hours). Empathy is critical with this population as the clinician is sometimes encouraging the patient to prioritize sleep above other activities such as engaging in the rest of the family's daytime activities.

However, many patients with phase delay problems benefit from simple sleep schedule modifications. For example, forcing a phase delayed patient to arise earlier and consistently, and removing stimulating substances (such as caffeine and text messaging at night) can have a profound impact. Adolescents are more complicated than adults to phase adjust due to their natural biorhythm to phase advance (discussed elsewhere in this chapter).

Medication warrants a brief note in this section. Two medications are marketed specifically for phase readjustment. One is melatonin, which is available over the counter, and the other is rozerem (Ramelteon), which is FDA approved for adults but not children. It is notable that there is no evidence that the use of stimulating drugs facilitates phase adjustment.[40] Rozerem and melatonin have the benefits of few side-effects and no known habit-forming risks. The clinician should take care of the timing at which either endogenous melatonin or bright light is administered based upon the phase response curve.

Circadian rhythm disorder and neurology

Though cognitive treatment of sleep disturbance is the focus of this chapter, it is noteworthy that as REM behavior disorder (RBD) is prominent in PD, melatonin has a low side-effect profile and has been used successfully to treat RBD.[42] It also has soporific benefits. The neurological disorders in which circadian rhythm is most problematic appear to be AD and PD.

Significant delays or advance to the timing of sleep may be a marker that a phase change is at the heart of the problem. Sundowning may be related to circadian misalignment (particularly in institutionalized patients who may be exposed to little natural light and have limited reasons to maintain a stable circadian schedule), and is an additional common problem which may be facilitated by light treatment. The suprachiasmatic nucleus (SCN), the circadian pacemaker, deteriorates in both the otherwise healthy aging and in patients with AD at a greater rate.[43] Brain lesions in the SCN and Meynert nucleus consequent to AD contribute to alterations in sleep homeostasis and circadian rhythms, as well as impairment of sleep-wake control.[43] This suggests that CRSD is likely secondary to the disease process itself in many patients. Both behavioral and pharmacological therapies may prove beneficial in these neurological disease states.

Conclusion

Insomnia and circadian rhythm disorders are prevalent in the general population. Behavioral treatment of these disorders involves the patient having the willingness and desire for change, as well as some understanding of how behavior, social pressures, and anxieties may be somatically manifested. As such, unlike many other sleep disorders, treatments require continuous patient participation, insight, and lifestyle change.

Neurological patients are disproportionately affected with sleep disturbance such as insomnia and circadian rhythm disorder compared with the general population. Facilitating change during the course of treatment is often difficult because of the patient's frustration with the sleep problem, burnout from multiple prior medical interventions for insomnia, and difficulty in divulging the range of personal issues and habits contributing to their distress. Through strategies used to treat insomnia, the doctor–patient relationship may also facilitate broader life changes and personal insights.

The first determination to be made is the magnitude to which behavior and psychological factors are at play in the symptom complaint. When cognitive behavioral interventions are indicated, the practitioner should take care to keep the patient involved in their treatment and to make sure the patient is in agreement with any intervention. In these patient populations, behavioral therapies may be the most effective form of treatment with fewer side-effects compared to pharmacological therapies.

References

1. Ancoli-Israel S, Roth T. Characteristics of insomnia in the United States: results of the 1991 National Sleep Foundation Survey. I. *Sleep* 1999; **22**(Suppl 2): S347–S353.

2. National Institutes of Health. State of the Science Conference statement on manifestations and management of chronic insomnia in adults, June 13–15, 2005. *Sleep* 2005; **28**: 1049–57.

3. Zammit GK, Weiner J, Damato N, Sillup GP, McMillan CA. Quality of life in people with insomnia. *Sleep* 1999; **22**(Suppl 2): S379–S385.

4. Daley M, Morin CM, LeBlanc M, Gregoire JP, Savard J, Baillargeon L. Insomnia and its relationship to health-care utilization, work absenteeism, productivity and accidents. *Sleep Med* 2009; **10**: 427–38.

5. Godet-Cayre V, Pelletier-Fleury N, Le Vaillant M, Dinet J, Massuel MA, Leger D. Insomnia and absenteeism at work. Who pays the cost? *Sleep* 2006; **29**: 179–84.

6. American Academy of Sleep Medicine. *International Classification of Sleep Disorders, Diagnostic and Coding Manual*, 2nd edn. Westchester, IL: American Academy of Sleep Medicine, 2005.

7. Attarian HP, Brown KM, Duntley SP, Carter JD, Cross AH. The relationship of sleep disturbances and fatigue in multiple sclerosis. *Arch Neurol* 2004; **61**: 525–8.

8. Ohayon MM, Roth T. Place of chronic insomnia in the course of depressive and anxiety disorders. *J Psychiatr Res* 2003; **37**: 9–15.

9. Buysse DJ, Angst J, Gamma A, Ajdacic V, Eich D, Rossler W. Prevalence, course, and comorbidity of insomnia and depression in young adults. *Sleep* 2008; **31**: 473–80.

10. Tsuno N, Besset A, Ritchie K. Sleep and depression. *J Clin Psychiatry* 2005; **66**: 1254–69.

11. Feige B, Al-Shajlawi A, Nissen C, et al. Does REM sleep contribute to subjective wake time in primary insomnia? A comparison of polysomnographic and subjective sleep in 100 patients. *J Sleep Res* 2008; **17**: 180–90.

12. Bonnet MH, Arand DL. Insomnia, metabolic rate and sleep restoration. *J Intern Med* 2003; **254**: 23–31.

13. Ferentinos P, Kontaxakis V, Havaki-Kontaxaki B, et al. Sleep disturbances in relation to fatigue in major depression. *J Psychosom Res* 2009; **66**: 37–42.

14. Morin CM, Vallieres A, Guay B, et al. Cognitive behavioral therapy, singly and combined with medication, for persistent insomnia: a randomized controlled trial. *JAMA* 2009; **301**: 2005–15.

15. Thase ME. Antidepressant treatment of the depressed patient with insomnia. *J Clin Psychiatry* 1999; **60**(Suppl 17): 28–31.

16. Perlis M, Gehrman P, Riemann D. Intermittent and long-term use of sedative hypnotics. *Curr Pharm Des* 2008; **14**: 3456–65.

17. Riemann D, Perlis ML. The treatments of chronic insomnia: a review of benzodiazepine receptor agonists and psychological and behavioral therapies. *Sleep Med Rev* 2009; **13**: 205–14.

18. Brajkovic L, Bras M, Milunovic V, et al. The connection between coping mechanisms, depression, anxiety and fatigue in multiple sclerosis. *Coll Antropol* 2009; **33**(Suppl 2): 135–40.

19. Figved N, Klevan G, Myhr KM, et al. Neuropsychiatric symptoms in patients with multiple sclerosis. *Acta Psychiatr Scand* 2005; **112**: 463–8.

20. Galeazzi GM, Ferrari S, Giaroli G, et al. Psychiatric disorders and depression in multiple sclerosis outpatients: impact of disability and interferon beta therapy. *Neurol Sci* 2005; **26**: 255–62.

21. Chahraoui K, Pinoit JM, Viegas N, Adnet J, Bonin B, Moreau T. [Alexithymia and links with depression and anxiety in multiple sclerosis]. *Rev Neurol Paris* 2008; **164**: 242–5.

22. Merlino G, Fratticci L, Lenchig C, et al. Prevalence of 'poor sleep' among patients with multiple sclerosis: an independent predictor of mental and physical status. *Sleep Med* 2009; **10**: 26–34.

23. Factor SA, McAlarney T, Sanchez-Ramos JR, Weiner WJ. Sleep disorders and sleep effect in Parkinson's disease. *Mov Disord* 1990; **5**: 280–5.

24. Young A, Home M, Churchward T, Freezer N, Holmes P, Ho M. Comparison of sleep disturbance in mild versus severe Parkinson's disease. *Sleep* 2002; **25**: 573–7.

25. Tandberg E, Larsen JP, Karlsen K. A community-based study of sleep disorders in patients

with Parkinson's disease. *Mov Disord* 1998; **13**: 895–9.

26. Stocchi F, Barbato L, Nordera G, Berardelli A, Ruggieri S. Sleep disorders in Parkinson's disease. *J Neurol* 1998; **245**(Suppl 1): S15–S18.

27. Dauvilliers Y. Insomnia in patients with neurodegenerative conditions. *Sleep Med* 2007; **8**(Suppl 4): S27–S34.

28. Morgenthaler T, Kramer M, Alessi C, et al. Practice parameters for the psychological and behavioral treatment of insomnia: an update. An American Academy of Sleep Medicine report. *Sleep* 2006; **29**: 1415–19.

29. Morin CM, Bootzin RR, Buysse DJ, Edinger JD, Espie CA, Lichstein KL. Psychological and behavioral treatment of insomnia: update of the recent evidence 1998–2004. *Sleep* 2006; **29**: 1398–414.

30. Bootzin RR. A Stimulus Control for Insomnia. *Proc Am Psychol Assoc* 1972; 395–6.

31. Spielman AJ, Caruso LS, Glovinsky PB. A behavioral perspective on insomnia treatment. *Psychiatr Clin North Am* 1987; **10**: 541–53.

32. Manber R, Edinger JD, Gress JL, San Pedro-Salcedo MG, Kuo TF, Kalista T. Cognitive behavioral therapy for insomnia enhances depression outcome in patients with comorbid major depressive disorder and insomnia. *Sleep* 2008; **31**: 489–95.

33. Edinger JD, Olsen MK, Stechuchak KM, et al. Cognitive behavioral therapy for patients with primary insomnia or insomnia associated predominantly with mixed psychiatric disorders: a randomized clinical trial. *Sleep* 2009; **32**: 499–510.

34. Carney CE, Waters WF. Effects of a structured problem-solving procedure on pre-sleep cognitive arousal in college students with insomnia. *Behav Sleep Med* 2006; **4**: 13–28.

35. Espie CA. *Overcoming Insomnia and Sleep Problems*, 2nd edn. London: Constable and Robinson, 2010.

36. National Heart, Lung, and Blood Institute Working Group on Insomnia. Insomnia: assessment and management in primary care. *Am Fam Physician* 1999; **59**: 3029–38.

37. Chesson AL, Anderson WM, Littner M, et al. Practice parameters for the nonpharmacologic treatment of chronic insomnia. *Sleep* 1999; **22**: 1128–33.

38. Carskadon MA, Labyak SE, Acebo C, Seifer R. Intrinsic circadian period of adolescent humans measured in conditions of forced desynchrony. *Neurosci Lett* 1999; **260**: 129–32.

39. Czeisler CA, Richardson GS, Coleman RM, et al. Chronotherapy: resetting the circadian clocks of patients with delayed sleep phase insomnia. *Sleep* 1981; **4**: 1–21.

40. Sack RL, Auckley D, Auger RR, et al. Circadian rhythm sleep disorders: part II, advanced sleep phase disorder, delayed sleep phase disorder, free-running disorder, and irregular sleep-wake rhythm. An American Academy of Sleep Medicine review. *Sleep* 2007; **30**: 1484–501.

41. Sack RL, Auckley D, Auger RR, et al. Circadian rhythm sleep disorders: part I, basic principles, shift work and jet lag disorders. *An American Academy of Sleep Medicine review. Sleep* 2007; **30**: 1460–83.

42. Boeve BF, Silber MH, Ferman TJ. Melatonin for treatment of REM sleep behavior disorder in neurologic disorders: results in 14 patients. *Sleep Med* 2003; **4**: 281–4.

43. Yesavage JA, Friedman L, Ancoli-Israel S, et al. Development of diagnostic criteria for defining sleep disturbance in Alzheimer's disease. *J Geriatr Psychiatry Neurol* 2003; **16**: 131–9.

10

Using Medications to Treat Insomnia

Andreea Andrei, MD

Menninger Department of Psychiatry and Behavioral Sciences, Baylor College of Medicine, The Methodist Hospital, USA

Introduction

What is sleep? A reversible behavioral state of perceptual disengagement from and unresponsiveness to the environment.

Why is sleep important? It provides a restorative, homeostatic function; sleep is involved in thermoregulation, energy conservation and consolidation of memories and recently learned associations of external stimuli and internal drives.

Sleep requirements

Length of sleep does not always correlate with a sleep disorder. There are the so-called "short sleepers", who need less than 6 hours of sleep per night and who are likely to be efficient, ambitious, socially adept, and content. At the other end of the spectrum, the "long sleepers" need more than 9 hours of sleep nightly; they tend to be mildly depressed, anxious, socially withdrawn. However, no matter what the baseline "need for sleep" is, sleep deprivation can have significant consequences for one's functioning; studies have shown that rats deprived of sleep have a debilitated appearance, with skin lesions and weight loss despite increased food intake; they have increased energy expenditure and decreased body temperature and all of these changes can lead up to death.[1]

Sleep architecture

Sleep is made up of two physiological states, non-rapid eye movement (NREM) and rapid eye movement (REM), that alternate in rhythmic fashion throughout the night, with a period of about 90 min.

Non-rapid eye movement sleep makes up about 75% of the entire sleep; it consists of a "idling brain in a movable body." It has four stages.

- Stage N1 (2–5%): light sleep
- Stage N2 (45–55%): leaves one moderately refreshed
- Stage N3 (15–20%): deep, slow-wave sleep

Rapid eye movement (REM) sleep/stage R makes up 25% of the entire sleep; during this time, we have a highly activated brain in a paralyzed body. Just as deep sleep restores the body, it is thought that REM sleep restores the mind. It provides energy to brain and body, supports daytime performance, and facilitates learning and memory. During REM, the brain is active and the most vivid dreams occur.

It now becomes easier to understand why good, restorative sleep is so important for human functioning.

Sleep disorders

When normal sleep is disrupted in terms of its quality, quantity, and/or timing, we talk about sleep disorders. There are various classifications of sleep disorders, including the *International Classification of Sleep Disorders* (ICSD, produced by the American Academy of Sleep Medicine) and the *Diagnostic and Statistical Manual of Mental Disorders* (DSM-IV, by the American Psychiatric Association). They are very detailed and exhaustive. For simplification purposes, we can think of sleep disorders as being:

- primary
- co-morbid, these being related to another mental disorder in contrast to being due to a general medical condition or substance related.

At any one moment 50% of adults are affected with one or more sleep problems.[2] Of these, insomnia is the most common complaint in the adult patient. Occasional insomnia is a fairly universal experience, while chronic insomnia occurs in about 10% of the population.

Insomnia

Insomnia is defined as complaints of disturbed sleep in the presence of adequate opportunity and circumstance for sleep; patients may experience difficulty in initiating sleep, difficulty in maintaining sleep or waking up too early. Non-restorative or poor-quality sleep has frequently been included in the definition, although there is controversy as to whether individuals with this complaint share similar pathophysiological mechanisms with the others. The ICSD defines insomnia as an almost nightly complaint of an insufficient amount of sleep or not feeling rested after the habitual sleep episode, despite adequate opportunity and circumstances for sleep. This is accompanied by worsened daytime functioning (fatigue; impairment in attention/memory/concentration; social or occupational dysfunction; mood disturbance or irritability; daytime sleepiness; decrease in motivation/energy/initiative; proneness for errors/accidents at work or while driving; tension, headaches or gastrointestinal symptoms; worries about sleep). Once the problem has lasted longer than 30 days, the patient is considered to have chronic insomnia.

The consequences of chronic insomnia can be significant: fatigue, impaired memory and cognitive functioning; overall lowered quality of life, with increased occupational dysfunction and decreased work performance.

Just like the other sleep disorders, insomnia can be primary or co-morbid. The term "co-morbid" rather than "secondary" is proposed,[3] due to the limited understanding of the mechanistic pathways in chronic insomnia. Rather frequently, insomnia is co-morbid with at least one other condition. Up to 90% of insomnia patients seen in primary care settings have co-morbid conditions.[4] Psychiatric problems are the most common conditions co-morbid with insomnia: 50% of those with chronic insomnia have a current psychiatric diagnosis or past psychiatric history. Two-thirds of patients referred to sleep disorder centers have a psychiatric disorder and more than half have a mood disorder.[5, 6] "Insomnia related to a mental disorder" was the most prevalent insomnia diagnosis assigned by sleep clinicians in a study involving five sleep centers.[6, 7]

✋ CAUTION

Once you suspect that a psychiatric co-morbidity exists, readily refer the patient for a psychiatric evaluation, not only to make sure that all psychiatric co-morbidities are diagnosed but also to avoid a potential misdiagnosis of bipolar depression for unipolar depression (while the clinical picture in an acute depressive episode is quite similar, the choice of medication is fundamentally different).

Co-morbidities include especially depression, anxiety, and substance use (including ethanol, street, and prescription drugs).

Insomnia can be a prodromal symptom or a risk factor for later development or recurrence of psychiatric disorder. Mood disorders (major depressive disorder, bipolar disorder) and anxiety disorders (generalized anxiety disorder, panic disorder, posttraumatic stress disorder) and insomnia are highly co-morbid, the relationship being bidirectional – depression can cause insomnia and insomnia can cause depression. The same holds true for anxiety and insomnia.

★ TIPS AND TRICKS

Sleep and psychiatric disorders (mainly depression, anxiety, substance use) are highly co-morbid, the relationship being bidirectional. Patients presenting with complaints of one must be assessed for the other.[8]

This high frequency of co-morbidity is particularly important when we think about treatment of insomnia. Accurate assessment and diagnosis of co-morbidities are essential for the appropriate treatment of insomnia. Combined treatment of both the mental disorder and the sleep disorder should be the standard of effective therapy for all patients.[10]

Treatment of insomnia (primary or co-morbid) consists of cognitive behavioral therapy for insomnia (CBT-I) and/or pharmacological treatment. It is generally believed that the improvement obtained through short-term pharmacological treatment does not continue after its discontinuation; however, CBT-I produces significant improvement of chronic insomnia in the short term and these improvements appear sustained at follow-up for up to 2 years.[11] Combined therapy (CBT-I plus medication) shows no consistent advantage or disadvantage over CBT-I alone. Comparisons with long-term pharmacotherapy are not available.[12]

This being said, there are a number of pharmacological options available for the treatment of insomnia. They tend to be used quite frequently and have some advantages over CBT-I: quicker onset of action, wider availability, and easier access to compared to treatment by certified behavioral sleep medicine therapists. Further information about CBT will be covered in Chapter 10.

Drugs used in treatment of insomnia

- Benzodiazepine receptor agonists (BzRA):
  - benzodiazepines (BZD)
  - non-benzodiazepines (non-BZD), the so-called "Z drugs"
- Ramelteon (Rozerem)
- Sedating antidepressants
- Antihistamines
- Other prescription drugs: atypical antipsychotics, gabapentin
- Other over-the-counter (OTC) agents: melatonin, valerian root

Benzodiazepine receptor agonists (BzRA)

Benzodiazepines can have widely variable half-lives and duration of action (there is no clear parallel between the two variables). The short- and medium-acting BZDs are preferred. In the list below, drugs in *italics* are FDA approved for insomnia treatment.

- Short-acting: alprazolam (Xanax, Xanax XR), *triazolam* (*Halcion*), midazolam
- Medium-acting: lorazepam (Ativan), *temazepam* (*Restoril*), estazolam (*ProSom*)
- Long-acting: diazepam (Valium), clonazepam (Klonopin), chlordiazepoxide (Librium), flurazepam (*Dalmane*)

Triazolam was the number one prescribed drug in the 1970s for insomnia.

The most commonly prescribed BZDs for insomnia treatment (including dosages) are:

- temazepam: 15–30 mg nightly; no adjustment for hepatic dysfunction
- triazolam: 0.25–0.5 mg nightly
- estazolam: 1–2 mg nightly
- flurazepam: 15–30 mg nightly
- quazepam : 7.5–15 mg nightly
- clonazepam: 1–2 mg nightly; beneficial especially in insomnia co-morbid with depression or restless legs syndrome (RLS); not FDA approved for insomnia.

> ★ TIPS AND TRICKS
>
> LOT (lorazepam-oxazepam-temazepam) is not hepatically metabolized, hence no dose adjustment is needed for hepatically impaired patients.

A few general points are worth keeping in mind about BZDs.

- Caution should be exercised when prescribing BZDs. While they are very useful when appropriately used, as a class they carry the potential for psychological and physiological dependence and addiction (higher risk with the short-acting ones). Always obtain a substance abuse history prior to prescribing a BZD; it is preferable to avoid using them in patients with prior history of alcohol or drug abuse.
- Even after only a few weeks of use, patients may experience withdrawal symptoms upon discontinuation, with rebound anxiety, tremor,

diaphoresis and even seizures and delirium; it is wise to taper them slowly (decrease by 10% per week).
- BZDs should be avoided during pregnancy and breastfeeding.
- They tend to be more effective when taken on an empty stomach.
- They carry the risk of daytime sedation, increased falls, cognitive impairment and confusion: these are worse for longer acting BZDs and in elderly people.
- They are highly protein bound but with no clinically significant displacement of other protein-bound drugs.
- They have no effect on cytochrome P450.
- Their metabolism is inhibited by cimetidine and some steroids, and accelerated in smokers.
- Most are very lipophilic.
- Elimination half-lives vary widely (higher in elderly people given their higher lipid-to-muscle ratio).
- Because of delayed accumulation and delayed elimination risk, daytime sedation, increased falls, and confusion, long half-life hypnotics are *not generally indicated*, especially for elderly people.

Z drugs

The Z drugs include:

- zolpidem (Ambien), also available in controlled-release (CR) formulation
- zaleplon (Sonata)
- eszopiclone (Lunesta).

Zolpidem (Ambien)

- Short-term treatment of sleep-onset insomnia; has been shown to decrease sleep latency for up to 35 days in controlled clinical studies; the CR formulation is also approved for sleep maintenance insomnia; the clinical trials performed in support of efficacy were up to 3 weeks (using polysomnography measurement up to 2 weeks in both adult and elderly patients) and 24 weeks (using patient-reported assessment in adult patients only) in duration.
- Preserves sleep stages (with only minor REM changes).
- On average, it prolongs total sleep 20–45 min or less; rarely makes early morning insomnia worse.

- Maximum dosage: adults 10 mg (or 12.5 mg extended release), elderly/debilitated/hepatic impairment 5 mg (or 6.25 mg extended release).
- Should not be taken with or immediately after a meal.
- To be taken immediately before bedtime.
- Withdrawal symptoms (mild dysphoria, insomnia, abdominal and muscle cramps, vomiting, diaphoresis, seizures) may occur with rapid dose reduction or discontinuation.

Zaleplon (Sonata)

- Short-term treatment of *sleep onset* insomnia; decreases time to sleep onset to up to 30 minutes; has not been shown to increase total sleep time or decrease number of awakenings.
- Adult dose 5–10 mg (maximum 20 mg) at bedtime; maximum 5 mg in elderly, debilitated, mild-to-moderate hepatic impairment. Recent recommendations from the United States Food and Drug Administration suggest that dosages for women be 5 mg given differences in drug metabolism between sexes.
- Avoid administration with high-fat meal.
- Half-life is approximately 1 hour.
- To be taken immediately before bedtime or after the patient has gone to bed and has experienced difficulty falling asleep.
- Mild rebound insomnia may occur with discontinuation; no significant withdrawal symptoms otherwise.

Eszopiclone (Lunesta)

- FDA approved for long-term use for sleep onset and maintenance insomnia.
- Likely to produce more hangover than zolpidem or zaleplon.
- Impairs morning digit symbol substitution compared to placebo.
- Same active ingredient as zopiclone, which has been associated with excess motor accidents in Europe.
- Maximum dosage 3 mg nightly (2 mg for elderly people).
- Taken immediately before bedtime and if 8 hours can be dedicated to sleep.

⚠ CAUTION

Careful reading of official prescribing information for eszopiclone as well as some published trials indicated that morning digit symbol substitution was impaired compared to placebo. Digit symbol substitution is one of the primary tasks used to test intelligence.

General notes on the Z drugs

- No effect on cytochrome P450; more specific for the alpha 1 subunit of the GABA A receptor, hence with sedating and amnestic properties similar to BZD, without the myorelaxant, anxiolytic, and anticonvulsant effect.
- It is questionable whether they produce any significant increase in the objective total sleep time for chronic insomnia.[14]

⚠ CAUTION

Uncommon side-effects of Z drugs include hallucinations, parasomnias including night eating or "zombie driving," nocturnal or early morning confusion. Patients should be warned about these potential side-effects.

General notes on the benzodiazepine receptor agonists

- Over age 60, risks seem to outweigh benefits, not only confusion and cognitive impairment but also falls.[15] However, there are some data suggesting that hypnotics in a nursing home population may reduce falls/injury (see Avidan AY, Fries BE, James ML. Insomnia and hypnotic use, recorded in the minimum data set, as predictors of falls and hip fractures in Michigan nursing homes. J Am Geriatr Soc. 2005 Jun; 53(6): 955–62.).
- Daytime impairment is much worse from hypnotics with a half-life longer than 4 hours. Risks from use of these drugs may include increased automobile accidents, falls, anterograde amnesia, and confusion. Because of its very short half-life, *zaleplon* probably does not cause daytime impairment, even when taken in the middle of the night. However, the clinical value of middle-of-the-night use of this drug has not been well demonstrated.

- Inconsistency between objective evidence of daytime impairment and subjective report of improved functioning.
- Risk of increasing depression.
- Risk of rebound insomnia, which may perpetuate the use of medication, as patients again experience insomnia upon stopping the medication.
- Regarding overdose, acute ingestion of benzodiazepine agonists alone rarely causes death, benzodiazepines combined with alcohol or other sedating drugs may be lethal, but barbiturates, ethchlorvynol, glutethimide, etc. may be much more lethal.
- Can be administered nightly versus intermittently (alternating 2–4 days at a time with and without medication) versus as needed.
- FDA class labeling after 2005 does not explicitly comment on the recommended duration of use.

Ramelteon (Rozerem)

- For sleep onset insomnia, clinical trials supported efficacy up to 6 months in duration.
- Melatonin agonist.
- Does not bind to benzodiazepine-GABA receptor: no cross-tolerance.
- Complex metabolism, active metabolites.
- Half life 1–2.6 hours (parent drug), 2–5 hours (metabolite).
- To be given 8 mg 30 min or less before bedtime.
- Not with or immediately after high-fat meal.
- Little benefit: appears to reduce sleep latency by 7–16 min, but has little value for maintaining sleep – similar to melatonin.
- Does *not* increase total sleep time substantially.
- Likely to have no risk of dependency and fewer other risks than benzodiazepine agonists.
- Potential side-effects include headaches, hallucinations, behavioral changes.
- Possible effects on reproductive endocrinology, e.g. prolactin, testosterone (could interfere with fertility or suppress testosterone).

Sedating antidepressants
Doxepine (Silenor)

- The only antidepressant which is FDA approved for the treatment of insomnia (though doxepin, the active ingredient of Silenor, is a tricyclic antidepressant at doses 10–100-fold higher than in Silenor).

- Indicated for sleep maintenance insomnia, with efficacy supported by clinical trials up to 3 months in duration.
- Used at rather low doses (3–6 mg nightly), where the antihistaminergic properties are predominant.
- To be taken 30 minutes or less before bedtime.
- Not to be taken within 3 hours of a meal, in order to minimize the potential for next-day effects.
- Contraindicated in untreated narrow angle glaucoma and severe urinary retention or if monoamine oxidase inhibitors have been taken within the last 2 weeks.
- Not associated with abuse/dependence/withdrawal/rebound insomnia.

Trazodone (Desyrel)

- Though not FDA approved for insomnia treatment, in 2005 trazodone was found to be the most commonly prescribed medication for treatment of insomnia in the United States.[3]
- Dose: 25–200 mg; low-adipose patients usually require less.
- Onset of action: 20–60 min; average peak level in 23 min.
- Though frequently used long term, there are no studies to show efficacy beyond 2 weeks.
- Effect on sleep stages: increases slow wave sleep; slight decrease in REM sleep.
- Advantages:
  - rapid onset of action
  - usually minimal or no tolerance develops
  - may be antidepressant or augment other antidepressants.
- Disadvantages:
  - hypotension, dizziness
  - daytime sedation ~20% of patients
  - gastrointestinal disturbance
  - risk of priapism in men (1:800 to 1:10,000)
  - cardiac rhythm risks, especially in elderly and patients with cardiac history.

> ♨ **CAUTION**
>
> Though commonly prescribed for insomnia, trazodone may not be appropriate in many patients, particularly in older adults or those with medical co-morbidities, given the cardiac risk.

Other antidepressants

- *Amitriptyline (Elavil)*: tricyclic antidepressant, most valuable when primarily treating another co-morbidity, such as chronic pain or migraine.
- *Mirtazapine (Remeron)*: though occasionally used, there are no data available to demonstrate its usefulness in management of chronic insomnia; however, when used for the treatment of depression, it may, through its antihistaminergic side-effects, have a positive impact on sleep.

Antihistamines

- Generally obtained by patients as over-the-counter medications, most include hydroxyzine (25–100 mg nightly), diphenhydramine (25–200 mg nightly) or doxylamine, by themselves or in combination with analgesics (such as Tylenol PM, Excedin PM, etc.).
- All types of antihistamines have a risk of negative effects on next-day functioning, with residual sedation and cognitive impairment, especially in the elderly who might also experience confusion or delirium. Also, via their anticholinergic properties, they may cause dry mouth, urinary retention, blurry vision, and increased intraocular pressure in people with narrow angle glaucoma.
- Onset of action 45 min–1 hours.
- Duration is variable, frequently longer than 8 hours.
- Decrease in REM sleep.
- Risk of habituation.
- REM rebound may occur on withdrawal, which can cause and/or worsen insomnia and can result in chronic use when acute treatment was planned.

> ♨ **CAUTION**
>
> Caution patients about the risk of regularly and excessively using OTC antihistamine-analgesic combinations; the analgesic component is likely to have significant and accumulating side-effects (e.g. gastrointestinal bleeding for non-steroidal antiinflammatory drugs, hepatic impairment for acetaminophen).

Other prescription drugs (used off label)

Atypical antipsychotics, such as quetiapine (Seroquel) or olanzapine (Zyprexa), are not recommended despite their rather common use in non-psychiatric settings; they carry significant risks, including but not limited to metabolic syndrome (including weight gain, hyperlipidemia, hyperglycemia, hypertension). These agents may play a role when treating insomnia due to a (hypo)manic episode, for example. Likewise, Seroquel XR, when used as adjunctive treatment for major depression, can be beneficial for the co-morbid insomnia; however, its use for insomnia alone is highly discouraged due to its heavy side-effects profile.

Gabapentin (Neurontin) may play a role when treating neuropathic pain co-morbid with insomnia; evidence of its efficacy in insomnia is too weak to justify its use otherwise.

Other over-the-counter agents

Melatonin

- Not FDA regulated, with high variability of strength between products, so hard to suggest efficacious dose.
- Some effect on sleep latency, though more likely to help as a chronobiotic (phase-shifting agent) than as a hypnotic.
- Believed to be fairly safe for short-term use.

Valerian root

- Small but consistent effect on sleep latency, with inconsistent effect on sleep continuity, sleep duration, and sleep architecture.
- Safety data are minimal, but there have been case reports of hepatotoxicity in persons taking herbal products containing valerian.[3]

Conclusion

An important side-effect to remember to talk about with your patients is the potential for abnormal thinking and behavioral changes that have been reported with sedatives/hypnotics. Complex behaviors like sleep-driving, preparing and eating food, making phone calls while not fully awake may occur after ingestion of the sedative/hypnotic, generally with amnesia for the event. Such side-effects can occur at therapeutic doses of medications,

though use of alcohol or other central nervous system depressants along with the sedative/hypnotics seems to increase the likelihood of such behaviors. Due to the risk to the patient and the community, discontinuation of the sedative/hypnotic should be strongly considered in patients who report a "sleep-driving" episode (or similar behaviors).

★ TIPS AND TRICKS

Patients may require education about the use of hypnotic agents. Patients should go to bed quickly after taking their hypnotic pill, should spend 8 hours in bed after taking a hypnotic, and should not mix hypnotics with use of alcohol or other drugs. In general, it is good practice to start dosages of hypnotic medications low and increase slowly, particularly in older patients or those who may metabolize the medications slowly.

So how is one supposed to choose from all the above choices, when it comes to treatment of insomnia? A number of factors should be taken into consideration in selecting an appropriate medication: symptom pattern, treatment goals, past treatment responses, patient preference, medication cost, availability of other treatments, co-morbid conditions, contraindications, concurrent medical interactions, and side-effects.[12]

The American Academy of Sleep Medicine clinical guidelines suggest the algorithm shown in Figure 10.1 for the treatment of chronic insomnia.

Pharmacological treatment of insomnia can be administered nightly versus intermittently (alternating 2–4 days at a time with and without medication) versus as needed. The post-2005 FDA labeling does not specifically address the recommended duration of treatment. Although in clinical practice these drugs are often effectively used for months at a time or even longer, a prudent approach is to reevaluate the need to continue using the medication every few weeks. As described above, various withdrawal symptoms (from rebound insomnia to anxiety or diaphoresis/seizures, depending on the particular medication) can occur after weeks of treatment; tapering off medications slowly reduces the risk of such withdrawal symptoms.

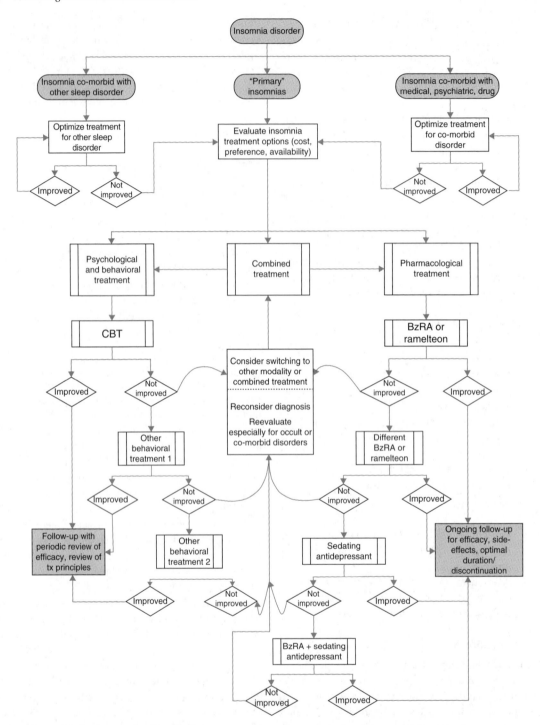

Figure 10.1 Algorithm for the treatment of chronic insomnia. Schutte-Rodin S, Broch L, Buysse D, Dorsey C, Sateia M. Clinical guideline for the evaluation and management of chronic insomnia in adults. *J Clin Sleep Med* 2008; **4**(5): 487–504.

References

1. Normal sleep and sleep disorders. In: Sadock B, Sadock V (eds) *Synopsis of Psychiatry*, 9th edn. Philadelphia: Lippincott Williams and Wilkins, 2003, pp756–82.
2. Worldwide project on sleep and health- WHO/MSA/MND/98.3.pg.3, World Health Organization publication, Geneva, 1998.
3. State-of-the-Science Conference on Manifestations and Management of Chronic Insomnia in Adults. *NIH Consensus and State-of-the-Art Statements* Volume 22, Number 2, June 13–15, 2005
4. Neubauer DN. Current and new thinking in the management of comorbid insomnia. *Am J Manage Care* 2009; **15**: S24–S32.
5. Tan TL, Kales JD, Kales A, et al. Biopsychobehavioral correlates of insomnia, IV: Diagnosis based on DSM-III. *Am J Psychiatry* 1984; **141**: 357–62.
6. Szelenberger W, Soldatos C. Sleep disorders in psychiatric practice. *World Psychiatry* 2005; **4**(3): 186–190.
7. Buysse DJ, Reynolds CF, Hauri PJ, et al. Diagnostic concordance for DSM-IV sleep disorders: a report from the APA/NIMH DSMIV trial. *Am J Psychiatry* 1994; **151**: 1351–60.
8. Peterson MJ, Benca RM. Sleep in mood disorders. *Sleep Med Clin* 2008; **3**: 231–49.
9. Mellman TA. Sleep and Anxiety Disorders. *Sleep Medicine Clinics* **3**(2008): 261–268
10. Sateia MJ. Update on sleep and psychiatric disorders. *Chest* 2009; **135**: 1370–9.
11. Morin C, Bootzin R, Buysse D, Edinger J, Espie C, Lichstein K. Psychological and behavioral treatment of insomnia: update of the recent evidence (1998–2004). *Sleep* 2006; **29**: 1398–414.
12. Schutte-Rodin S, Broch L, Buysse D, Dorsey C, Sateia M. Clinical guideline for the evaluation and management of chronic insomnia in adults. *J Clin Sleep Med* 2008; **4**(5): 487–504.
13. Krystal AD, Walsh JK, Laska E, et al. Sustained efficacy of eszopiclone over 6 months of nightly treatment: results of a randomized, double-blind, placebo-controlled study in adults with chronic insomnia. *Sleep* 2003; **26**(7): 793–9.
14. Buscemi N, Vandermeer B, Friesen C, et al. The efficacy and safety of drug treatments for chronic insomnia in adults: a meta-analysis of RCTs. *J Gen Intern Med* 2007; **22**: 1335–50.
15. Glass J, Lanctot KL, Herrmann N, Sproule BA, Busto UE. Sedative hypnotics in older people with insomnia: meta-analysis of risks and benefits. *BMJ* 2005; **331**(7526): 1169.

11

Parasomnias: Diagnosis, Evaluation, and Treatment

Douglas B. Kirsch, MD, FAASM

Harvard Medical School and Division of Sleep Neurology, Department of Neurology, Brigham and Women's Hospital, USA

Types of parasomnias

The word parasomnia derives from Greek: *para* (along with) and Latin: *somnus* (sleep). Parasomnias are defined clinically as "undesirable physiological phenomena which occur during entry into sleep, within sleep, or during arousals from sleep."[1] These behaviors are typically complex and can range from being inconvenient or embarrassing for patients to potentially causing severe injury to themselves or to a bed partner. The most basic brain states may be represented during some of these behaviors; many actions are related to locomotion, food, aggression, and sex. During a parasomnia, the patient does not have conscious volitional control of the behavior, so the actions that occur are considered legally an automatism. Thus, a patient is typically not considered legally liable for actions that occur during a parasomnia.

This chapter will review the common parasomnias, discuss methods of evaluation, and examine different treatment modalities. In patients with parasomnias, physicians need to consider alternative diagnoses, including both other sleep disorders and non-sleep medical or psychiatric disorders, and assess patients completely so as to avoid incorrect management. The parasomnias are categorized into rapid eye movement (REM), non-REM (NREM), and Other parasomnias (Table 11.1); this chapter will review each in turn.

The pathogenesis of parasomnias is not fully understood. It appears that there is an oscillation between the sleep state and wake state that leads to some aspects of each state being interwoven. This dissociation of sleep stages results in the overlapping of wakefulness and NREM sleep (confusional arousals, somnambulism, and night terrors) or wakefulness and REM sleep (REM sleep behavior disorder). Sleep environment, other sleep disorders, and individual genetics contribute to the likelihood of having a parasomnia. Other factors, such as intense physical activity, fever, sleep deprivation, and medications (neuroleptics, central nervous system depressants), increase the chances of parasomnia occurrence.

NREM parasomnias

Typically, NREM parasomnias occur in children and the behaviors happen in the first half of the nocturnal sleep period, when slow-wave sleep is more prominent. NREM parasomnias are less commonly present in the adult population but they should not be discounted when the history supports the diagnosis. A family history of abnormal nocturnal behaviors is often present in patients presenting with a clear parasomnia.

Confusional arousals typically occur upon arousal from slow-wave (stage N3) sleep or when nearing wakefulness in the morning. Patients with confusional arousals, who are more commonly children than adults, tend to be disoriented during the behavior with slow speech, poor cognition, and no memory for the event in the morning. During the event, particularly during a forced awakening, behavior may be clearly unacceptable and

Sleep Medicine in Neurology, First Edition. Edited by Douglas B. Kirsch.
© 2014 John Wiley & Sons, Ltd. Published 2014 by John Wiley & Sons, Ltd.

Table 11.1 Categories of parasomnias

Category	Subcategory
NREM parasomnias (disorders of arousal)	Confusional arousals Sleepwalking Sleep terrors
REM parasomnias	REM sleep behavior disorder Recurrent isolated sleep paralysis Nightmare disorder
Other parasomnias	Sleep-related dissociative disorders Sleep enuresis Sleep-related groaning (catathrenia) Exploding head syndrome Sleep-related hallucinations Sleep-related eating disorder Parasomnias, unspecified Parasomnias due to drugs or substance Parasomnias due to medical condition

NREM, non-rapid eye movement; REM, rapid eye movement.

potentially violent. The behaviors generally last a few minutes but in rare cases may last up to hours. In children aged 3–13 years old, the prevalence of confusional arousal has been reported at 17% whereas in adults older than 15 years old, the prevalence is 3–4%. Sexsomnia, or sexual activities occurring during sleep, typically seen in adults, are likely a subtype of confusional arousal.

Ambulating during sleep or sleepwalking is also a common parasomnia, occurring in up to 17% of children, peaking at 8–12 years of age. Episodes may range from routine behaviors to those more inappropriate (urinating into trashcans or climbing out a window) and may be violent in rare cases, particularly when someone tries to awaken the patient. Amnesia for the nocturnal event is typical in both children and adults. There is a strong genetic association as this type of parasomnia runs in families. Generally, sleepwalking can be considered normal in childhood, unless there are clinical consequences; if it continues

after adolescence or begins in adulthood, an evaluation should occur.

> ☝ **CAUTION**
>
> Sleepwalking patients should typically be redirected back to bed calmly and quietly, unless the patient's safety is at risk. Attempting to awaken the patient from their parasomnia may result in confusion, agitation, and rarely violence.

Sleep terrors may be difficult to distinguish from sleepwalking in adults, as they consist of arousal from slow-wave sleep, often a piercing scream, as well as high autonomic discharge and behavioral manifestations of fear. Patients may run suddenly out of bed and in some cases may be violent. Young patients (age 4–12), in whom the condition is much more common, may be amnestic for the events; older patients may have dream fragments that are remembered in association with the behavior. While in young children, this disorder is not clearly linked to psychopathology, there is some evidence suggesting a link between sleep terrors and psychiatric conditions in adults.

REM parasomnias

Rapid eye movement behavior disorder (RBD) occurs when a patient has abnormal behaviors during REM sleep, a typical period of atonia, in combination with sleep disruption. Injuries to self or a bed partner are commonly reported in this disorder, as the episodes are typically associated with violent dream enactment. Flailing, punching, kicking, and shouting are common, but leaving the bed is less common. Episodes more typically occur in the second half of the night, when a larger percentage of the night is REM sleep. This disorder may be idiopathic but can occur in the setting of withdrawal from alcohol, drug intoxication, and during use of certain medications (see Parasomnias due to Drugs or Substance). RBD is a male-dominated diagnosis that has been connected to many neurological conditions. Most notably, RBD may predate other symptoms of an alpha-synucleinopathy by many years; two-thirds of men over 50 diagnosed with RBD developed a parkinsonian disorder at a mean interval of 13 years from the RBD diagnosis (see

Chapter 13 for further details). Other neurological disorders which may have RBD as a symptom include narcolepsy, ischemic and hemorrhagic strokes, multiple sclerosis, and brainstem tumors.

✋ CAUTION

RBD can be a dangerous condition, for both the patient and bed partner. If safety is a concern for the bed partner, an alternative sleeping location should be suggested until treatment is effective. If patients are prone to leaving the bed, a bed alarm may be helpful. The bedroom safety should be maximized and if the patient is prone to leaving the bed, the windows should be protected and sharp edges in the bedroom should be minimized.

Recurrent isolated sleep paralysis often provokes anxiety in patients, at least initially, but carries no risk of harm to the patient. This parasomnia can occur either at sleep onset or when awakening from sleep and may be associated with visual, auditory or tactile hallucinations. The prevalence is likely between 15–40% for at least one episode of sleep paralysis over the lifespan; the recurrent form of this disorder commonly begins in adolescence. Episodes are more likely to occur in the setting of sleep deprivation or irregular sleep schedules. This disorder may have a genetic mechanism; maternal transmission is suspected. The mechanism is likely the intrusion of REM sleep phenomena (atonia, dream-like hallucinations) into the wake state.

Nightmare disorder occurs when recurrent nightmares (disturbing mental experiences, typically occurring during REM sleep) disrupt sleep abruptly. These dreams are often vivid and can be recalled in great detail; nightmares are distinguished from "bad dreams" by the nightmare provoking an awakening from sleep. Nightmares are a common experience; approximately 75% of children remember a nightmare over the course of their childhood and 50–85% of adults report having an occasional nightmare. A much smaller number of adults (2–8%) report current problems with nightmares; posttraumatic stress disorder (PTSD) may play a role in a large portion of these cases. Cases of nightmares tend to decrease with aging, though some older adults will continue to report them.

Table 11.2 Differentiating NREM Parasomnias and REM Sleep Behavior Disorder

	NREM	REM
Typical timing	First half of the night	Second half of the night
Typical age	Children and young adults	Older adults
Memory for the behavior	Often limited	Generally good
Gender	Can be either	More often male than female

NREM, non-rapid eye movement; REM, rapid eye movement.

Interestingly, polysomnography during intense nightmares may demonstrate little autonomic change.

Differentiating between NREM parasomnias and REM sleep behavior disorder may at times be difficult based on history alone. Some useful tips are given in Table 11.2.

Other parasomnias

Sleep-related dissociative disorders involve "disruption in the usually integrated functions of the consciousness, memory, identity or perception of the environment." Three DSM-IV dissociative disorders have been observed in the nocturnal context: dissociative identity disorder, dissociative fugue, and dissociative disorder not otherwise specified. Most patients with these disorders have corresponding daytime symptoms and often have a prior history of physical or sexual abuse. The episodes occur during clear electroencephalograph (EEG) wakefulness either in wake-sleep transitions or upon clear awakenings from sleep.

Sleep enuresis, or bedwetting, does not occur as a disorder until at least the age of 5 years old in which wetting episodes occur at least twice per week. Primary enuresis occurs when a child has never been dry at night for at least 6 months; secondary occurs when the patient has been dry for at least 6 months and then begins having wetting episodes at least twice per week for at least 3 months. Prevalence of primary enuresis categorized by age is shown in Table 11.3. Secondary enuresis in a child may occur in patients who have undergone significant psychosocial stresses; in an adult, it may be related to

Table 11.3 Primary sleep enuresis prevalence

Age (years)	% with primary enuresis
4	30%
6	10%
7	7%
10	5%
12	3%
18	1–2%

Adapted from *International Classification of Sleep Disorders*, 2nd edn.

diabetes, urinary tract infection (UTI), obstructive sleep apnea (OSA), and epilepsy.

Catathrenia (or sleep-related groaning) is typically a nightly disorder in which expiratory groaning occurs during REM sleep, often in clusters. The disorder is associated with bradypnea but neither respiratory distress nor abnormal motor activity. The behavior is usually reported by a housemate or bed partner, though the patient may be unaware of it and may have no sleep complaint. The disorder is rare, reportedly occurring in 0.5% of 1836 consecutive sleep studies at a multidisciplinary sleep center.

Exploding head syndrome is "characterized by a sudden loud imagined noise or a sense of a violent explosion in the head occurring as the patient is falling asleep or waking during the night."[1] Some examples of the noise include a painless loud bang or a clash of cymbals, though not all the noises are alarming. Associated with the event is a sense of fright and some patients suspect that they are having a stroke. The events may be variable in frequency up to several times per night and may occur in clusters. The syndrome can occur in a wide age range and has a benign course with no evident sequelae other than occasional insomnia.

Sleep-related hallucinations are typically visual experiences occurring at the onset of sleep (hypnogogic) or upon awakening (hypnopompic). Other types of hallucinations may include auditory, tactile or kinetic. Hypnogogic hallucinations are more commonly reported than hypnopompic ones. An association with sleep paralysis is sometimes observed. Hallucinations are more common in adolescents and young adults and appear to reduce in frequency with aging. Prevalence is 25–37% for hypnogogic and 7–13% for hypnopompic hallucinations.

The majority of events evaluated in studies were related to REM sleep, though a few of the events were NREM associated.

Sleep-related eating disorder (SRED) involves recurrent episodes of involuntary eating and drinking occurring during arousals from sleep with negative consequences. The SRED episodes may occur at any time during the night. The episodes are typically only partially recalled, though some patients may have clear recall. Patients may eat peculiar foods or consume inedible or toxic substances during the episodes, generally not eating foods preferred during daytime hours, and may perform dangerous behaviors in trying to obtain or prepare food. Effects of the disorder may include insomnia (from sleep disruption), sleep-related injury (burns, lacerations), morning anorexia, and weight gain. The disorder typically occurs in females more than males and may be more prevalent in patients with eating disorders. This disorder may be a sleepwalking variant and may be associated with other sleep disorders and/or use of medications (such as zolpidem or psychotropic medications).

> ★ TIPS AND TRICKS
>
> SRED may need to be distinguished from nocturnal eating syndrome (NES). NES criteria consist of consumption of 50% or more of daily calories after the evening meal, eating after waking from sleep, and morning anorexia. NES is typically considered an eating disorder, not a sleep disorder, due to the patient's clear awareness of their eating activities at night compared to those patients with SRED. There is ongoing debate about the relationship between these two disorders.

Unspecified parasomnias is a temporary diagnosis, solely for use when the type of parasomnia is not easily classifiable or there is a strong suspicion of an undiagnosed psychiatric condition as the cause for the parasomnia.

Parasomnia due to drug or substance requires a close temporal relationship between exposure to the substance and the onset of symptoms. Parasomnias related to medications may arise out of either NREM or REM sleep. Some of the medications which have been previously described as triggering RBD are given in Table 11.4. Withdrawal from alcohol or drugs (e.g. cocaine, amphetamine) may also cause RBD symptoms.

Parasomnias due to a medical condition require an underlying medical or neurological cause of the parasomnia. The most common example of this disorder is in RBD, which may arise as part of a synuncleinopathy as noted above. Agrypnia excitata is a condition which includes dream enactment as part of its varied symptoms (generalized motor overactivity, loss of slow-wave sleep, autonomic sympathetic activation), and which may occur in the setting of delirium tremens or fatal familial insomnia. Sleep-related visual hallucinations occur in patients with narcolepsy, Parkinson's disease, dementia with Lewy bodies, and visual loss (Charles–Bonnet hallucinations).

Evaluation of the patient with a parasomnia

History

Good clinical history taking is important when evaluating a patient with a parasomnia. Observers of the behavior as well as the patient should be queried about aspects of their nocturnal behavior. The history alone in many cases can guide the clinician to an appropriate diagnosis and a potential treatment. Some useful questions in the evaluation of a parasomnia are listed in Table 11.5.

To clarify the questions in Table 11.5, NREM parasomnias tend to occur in the first half of the night. Patients are unlikely to recall dreams associated with NREM behaviors (also often not recalling the behavior if asked about it afterward); REM-related parasomnias are more likely to happen in the latter half of the sleep period and are often associated with vivid dreaming which may at least partially match the patient's behaviors.

Attempting to differentiate seizures and parasomnias can be difficult based on clinical history alone, though certain aspects may guide further testing. Seizures tend to be stereotyped (though some seizure subtypes may be less stereotyped) and tongue biting and incontinence may be associated

Table 11.4 Selected medications which may trigger RBD

Selective serotonin reuptake inhibitors
Venlafaxine
Tricyclic antidepressants
Monoamine oxidase inhibitors
Mirtazapine
Bisoprolol
Selegiline
Cholinergic treatments (for Alzheimer's disease)

Adapted from *International Classification of Sleep Disorders*, 2nd edn.

Table 11.5 Diagnostic questions regarding nocturnal behaviors

General questions	What behaviors occur during the night?
	How long have they been occurring?
	How many nights per month/week does the behavior occur?
	How many times per night does the behavior occur?
	Has the behavior been associated with injuries to the patient or bed partner?
	Are there signs of other sleep disorders (snoring, gasping, leg movements)?
	Does anyone else in the family have similar symptoms?
	Is the behavior associated with any medications use or substance use?
NREM versus REM	Does the behavior tend to occur in the first half or the second half of the night?
	Is the behavior associated with dream enactment?
Seizure versus parasomnia	Is the behavior stereotyped?
	Is tongue biting or incontinence associated with the behavior?
	Does the patient have a prior history of seizure?
	Does the patient have memory of the behaviors?

NREM, non-rapid eye movement; REM, rapid eye movement.

with certain seizure subtypes. A history of prior seizures suggests a higher likelihood of a seizure causing the nocturnal behavior. Though for many seizures and most parasomnias, the patient's memory of the behavior is limited, in cases of some nocturnal frontal lobe seizures, memory of the event may be preserved. Further discrimination of seizures and parasomnias will be detailed below.

Physical examination

The physical examination is infrequently useful in the evaluation of parasomnia patients as the patients typically do not have abnormal findings. As obstructive sleep apnea at times may elicit parasomnias or increase their frequency, an evaluation of the patient's risk for sleep-disordered breathing should be performed. To do this, physicians should evaluate Body Mass Index, neck circumference, jaw shape, and size of the orophayrynx. Neurological examination may offer further information when assessing the risk for an underlying seizure disorder; asymmetries in the motor, sensory or reflex examination or other abnormalities suggesting a central nervous system pathology could point toward an underlying source of seizures. Though some physicians have viewed parasomnias as being linked to psychiatric disorders, the data supporting this link are currently unclear. A full psychiatric evaluation may not be necessary unless prompted by other symptoms or underlying history.

Parasomnia identification and initial testing

Initial assessment

The history and examination of the patient help distinguish between the many causes of nocturnal behaviors. Home videos, if present, may also be useful in the initial evaluation. Videos of the behavior allow the clinician to better understand the behavior and to gauge the timing of the event during the night and thus help in correct categorization of the parasomnia.

Often a good clinical history (noted above) can aid differentiation between NREM and REM parasomnias. As indicated previously, as REM sleep comprises a larger percentage of the second half of the night than the first, REM-related parasomnias tend to occur in the latter half of the night. In addition, dream enactment occurs, in which the

Table 11.6 Elements of patient history suggesting seizure

Prior seizure history
Stereotypical behavior
Specific dystonic posturing
Tongue biting and/or incontinence
Behaviors which are not complex or directed
May occur at any time of night
Confusion after the behavior
Known brain lesion

patient will remember a vivid dream upon awakening from an episode, while the bed partner describes the patient performing behaviors similar to the activity of that dream while asleep. Anecdotally, REM-related behaviors often have a phasic or "jerky" appearance and speech occurring during the episode may be semi-coherent or unintelligible.

A common difficulty in assessing nocturnal behaviors is determining if a seizure may be the primary cause. Historical elements that might suggest a seizure include the elements seen in Table 11.6.

Though many types of seizures exist, the most difficult to distinguish from parasomnias are nocturnal frontal lobe seizures. Frontal lobe seizures are often difficult to visualize on surface EEG leads and are associated with very complex behaviors. This seizure subtype may be sleep specific, without evident waking episodes, and in some cases may have autosomal dominant genetic transmission. Though parasomnias may also be transmitted through families, the genetics is less clear. Given the difficulty in distinguishing certain parasomnias from seizures by history, diagnostic testing may be the most efficient route of determining the origins of a behavior if the history alone is not sufficient.

Routine EEG

Most parasomnias do not require a routine daytime EEG as part of the initial work-up. If the patient's nocturnal behavior appears potentially seizure related, a sleep-deprived EEG performed during wake and sleep may be useful in ascertaining whether any abnormal electrical brain activity occurs. It is important to evaluate sleep on the EEG when assessing a potential parasomnia, as sleep may be an activator of certain types of epileptic activity. The potential yield of the EEG may be increased with a longer recording time than the typical 30 minutes, though this option is not always available. It is important to remember that a small percentage of the population will have an abnormal EEG, but the abnormality may not be linked to a seizure disorder.

Polysomnography for parasomnias

American Academy of Sleep Medicine (AASM) guidelines state that in the case of "typical, uncomplicated, and non-injurious parasomnias when the diagnosis is clearly delineated," polysomnography is not indicated.[2] Thus, a polysomnogram is unnecessary for most cases of typical disorders of arousal, nightmares, enuresis, sleep talking, and bruxism. Similarly, patients who have seizures but no sleep complaints do not routinely require an overnight study. However, there are several reasons to pursue a polysomnogram for patients with abnormal nocturnal behaviors in the case of a normal initial work-up (see Table 11.7).

Testing in the sleep laboratory should occur for violent or potentially injurious nocturnal behaviors. With the goals of preventing harm to the patient or another individual, an accurate diagnosis and plan for intervention are paramount. Additionally, in cases when a patient is involved in a situation with legal implications, a polysomnogram may minimize diagnostic uncertainty and clarify the forensic situation. For patients with a likely seizure disorder and a negative routine EEG or those with an atypical parasomnia (based on the description of the event, the age when the behaviors began, or highly stereotypical nature), performing an overnight sleep study may elucidate the specific diagnosis. Lastly, polysomnography should be arranged for situations in which conventional treatment of parasomnias or nocturnal seizures disorders occurs but does not resolve the patient's symptoms.

In cases where a routine EEG does not demonstrate an epileptogenic appearance but seizure remains high on the differential diagnosis, the next step should be to undertake a polysomnogram with additional derivations. Electromyography (EMG) channels are typically placed on the anterior tibialis; additional EMG leads can be positioned on the arms

Table 11.7 Reasons to pursue polysomnography in assessment of parasomnias

1. To assist with the diagnosis of paroxysmal arousals or other sleep disruptions that are thought to be seizure related when the initial clinical evaluation and results of a standard EEG are inconclusive
2. In evaluating sleep-related behaviors that are violent or otherwise potentially injurious to the patient or others
3. When evaluating patients with sleep behaviors suggestive of parasomnias that are unusual or atypical because of the patient's age at onset; the time, duration, or frequency of occurrence of the behavior; or the specifics of the particular motor patterns in question (e.g. stereotypical, repetitive, or focal)
4. In situations with forensic considerations (e.g. if onset follows trauma or if the events themselves have been associated with personal injury)
5. When the presumed parasomnia or sleep-related seizure disorder does not respond to conventional therapy
6. When there is a strong suspicion of an underlying sleep disorder, such as obstructive sleep apnea
7. With a strong history of REM sleep behavior disorder, in order to ensure a correct diagnosis and the absence of an underlying secondary sleep disorder

Data from Kushida CA, Littner MR, Morgenthaler T et al. Practice parameters for the indications for polysomnography and related procedures: an update for 2005. Sleep 2005; 28: 499–521.

(extensor digitorum) for more accurate assessment of movements during sleep. The standard EEG montage for polysomnography requires leads unilaterally on the frontal region (F3), central region (C3), and occipital region (O1); back-up leads are placed on the contralateral side (F4, C4, O2).[3] When seizures appear a likely cause of the abnormal nocturnal behavior, additional EEG leads may be useful. In a limited extra EEG montage setting, bilateral temporal leads provide coverage over a brain area prone to seizure genesis; however, in centers with the appropriate technology and training, a polysomnogram with a full-head EEG (16 leads) in the 10–20 system is preferred. This study type requires a sleep medicine practitioner who is at ease with interpretation of EEG signals, most often a neurologist or a physician who has undergone specialty training in EEG or epilepsy. These expanded studies take much longer to interpret than a standard polysomnogram, as full-head EEG signals are typically examined in 10-second epochs (compared to 30 second or more for polysomnography). Advances in technology, such as automated spike detection software, may speed the interpretation, though these programs may not provide a full analysis of the non-spike EEG waveforms.

Video monitoring is considered part of polysomnography but in the case of an abnormal sleep-related behavior, the technologists and physicians should have access to video and audio with appropriate clarity. In some cases, small movements by the patient guide the sleep medicine specialist to a brain location that may be abnormal. The video needs to be synchronized to the EEG data, so that any behavior can be well correlated with brain wave changes. Sleep technologists are trained to closely document all observable behaviors when monitoring these patients as well as to ask patients questions during and after the nocturnal behaviors to assess their cognitive state.

A single overnight full-head EEG polysomnogram may not always finalize a diagnosis. A negative study, with a history solidly suggestive of seizure, may require repetition at a future time. Additionally, for patients who have a high likelihood of seizure activity or otherwise requiring a complete diagnosis with previously negative expanded polysomnography, long-term monitoring in a comprehensive epilepsy unit should be strongly considered.

The algorithm (Figure 11.1)

As suggested earlier in this chapter, the clinical history and examination should guide decision making regarding testing. For suspected seizures, routine EEG and expanded polysomnography with full-head EEG should be considered, while in difficult-to-diagnose cases, long-term in-hospital epilepsy monitoring may be necessary. For suspected parasomnias, determination of the most likely type of parasomnia is the best guide to treatment. In addition, if an underlying non-parasomnia sleep disorder is suspected, evaluation by polysomnography and appropriate treatment of that disorder may

limit or cure nocturnal abnormal behaviors. Violent or potentially injurious parasomnias as well as most REM-related parasomnias may require polysomnography to ensure the correct diagnosis and to aid in treatment recommendations. In all cases of parasomnias potentially leading to injury of the patient or others in the house, strong safety recommendations to the patient and family should be reviewed.

Treatment of parasomnias

In most cases, parasomnias are not dangerous, are unlikely to cause significant injury, and have minimal daytime impact. However, as mentioned above, in some cases, they may have severe consequences, including bodily injury and death. As with any treatment, weighing side-effect versus benefit is of paramount importance. With many parasomnias, particularly NREM parasomnias in children, no treatment is necessary, as the risks to the child are low and generally the only effect of the behavior is parental sleep deprivation.

Reviewing good sleep habits, treating other sleep disorders, and ensuring an optimal and safe sleeping environment often help minimize parasomnias at any age and potential injury to the patient. Treatment of other sleep disorders (such as obstructive sleep apnea or restless legs syndrome) and other medical disorders likely to disrupt sleep (such as gastroesophageal reflux disease or nocturia) is likely to minimize coincident parasomnias. Use of alcohol or illicit drugs may increase risk of a nocturnal behavior occurring.

Generally speaking, patients in the midst of a NREM parasomnia should not be interfered with or restrained unless risk of injury is imminent; gentle redirection may be useful in some cases. Scheduled awakenings just prior to the usual time of the parasomnia may prevent the behavior from occurring. Use of bed alarms may awaken the patient or alert family members to the behavior to help minimize injury to the patient. In some cases of patients with NREM parasomnias (e.g. confusional arousals, sleepwalking), psychological techniques such as relaxation training and hypnosis have been used with some positive benefit (Box 11.1).

In cases of frequent, dangerous or difficult-to-treat NREM parasomnias which have not responded to conservative treatment, pharmacological options should be considered. Most commonly, benzodiaz-

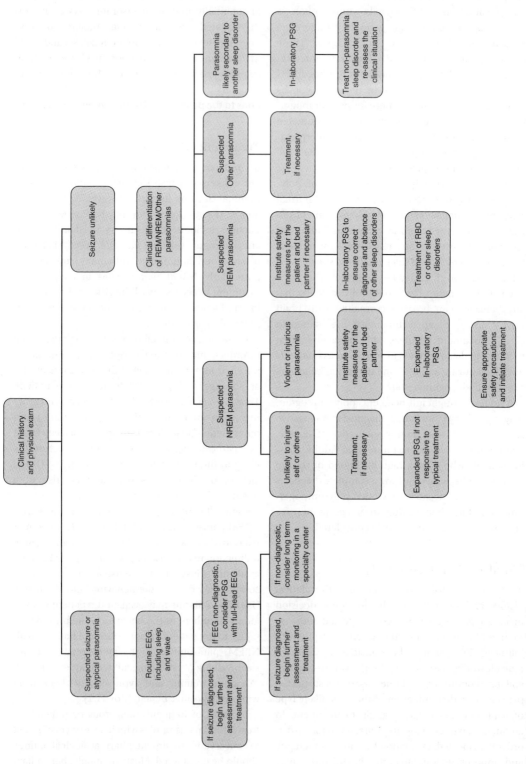

Figure 11.1 Parasomnia algorithm.

Box 11.1 Potential interventions for parasomnia treatment beyond direct pharmacological management

Keep a stable sleep schedule, going to bed and getting up at the same time

Aim for adequate nightly sleep (typically 7.5–8 hour/night for adults, more for children)

Maintain a good sleeping environment (i.e. avoid stimuli that may disrupt sleep – noises, light, etc.)

Minimize stress during waking hours

Treat non-parasomnia sleep disorders (OSA, restless legs syndrome, etc.)

Treat medical symptoms that may disrupt sleep (acid reflux, pain, nocturia)

Avoid ongoing use of substances which may increase parasomnia risk, including some hypnotic medications (such as zolpidem), alcohol, and illicit drugs

epines are used, given a history of effectiveness with a low side-effect profile. The choice of benzodiazepine should be in part driven by the timing of episodes: shorter-acting benzodiazepines for episodes which occur primarily in the beginning of the night, longer-acting benzodiazepines for episodes which occur later in the night or which are less predictable. Possible options for NREM parasomnias might include triazolam 0.125–0.5 mg, zolpidem 5–10 mg, lorazepam 1–2 mg, and clonazepam 0.5–2 mg. Sleep-related eating syndrome may respond best to different medications depending on the patient's history or coincident symptoms, including benzodiazepines, selective serotonin reuptake inhibitors, topiramate, or dopamine agonists.

With regard to REM sleep behavior disorder, if there is not a clear cause (OSA or other cause of sleep fragmentation), then medication is typically indicated if there is any sign of risk to the patient or bed partner. Clonazepam is frequently chosen as the primary form of treatment, in a similar dosing pattern to that seen for NREM parasomnias (0.5–2 mg); lorazepam (1–2 mg) is an alternative choice. These medications may not rid the patient of the abnormal muscle activity during REM sleep, but may reduce arousals during sleep leading to

complex behaviors. Melatonin demonstrates some efficacy in RBD control and has few, if any, side-effects. Treatment doses for melatonin range from 3 to 12 mg, though as it is not well regulated in the United States some caution should be used; bottle dosage amounts may not well reflect actual pill content. Finally, many other medications have been reportedly effective in small case studies or case reports, including imipramine, carbamazepine, and dopamine-promoting drugs (including carbidopa-levodopa and dopamine agonists, such as pramipexole and ropinirole). A recent AASM practice parameter (2010) has described the data on medication treatments of RBD in detail.[4]

Conclusion

Complex behaviors which occur during sleep are often challenging to diagnose and treat. It is imperative to obtain a good history, including video documentation at home if possible. In-laboratory polysomnography is not required for diagnosis of some parasomnias, but may be necessary in specific cases, particularly when trying to differentiate parasomnias from seizures or evaluate potentially injurious nocturnal behaviors. Treatment of parasomnias is quite dependent on making a correct diagnosis; both pharmacological and non-pharmacological options exist. In many patients with parasomnias, no treatment is needed; more aggressive treatment is typically necessary only for cases with the potential for morbidity or mortality.

References

1. American Academy of Sleep Medicine. *International Classification of Sleep Disorders, Diagnostic and Coding Manual*, 2nd edn. Westchester, IL: American Academy of Sleep Medicine, 2005.
2. Kushida CA, Littner MR, Morgenthaler T, et al. Practice parameters for the indications for polysomnography and related procedures: an update for 2005. *Sleep* 2005; **28**(4): 499–521.
3. Iber C, Ancoli-Israel S, Chesson A, Quan SF for the American Academy of Sleep Medicine. *The AASM Manual for the Scoring of Sleep and Associated Events: Rules, Terminology and Technical Specifications*. Westchester, IL. American Acadmey of Sleep Medicine, 2007.

4. Aurora RN, Zak RS, Maganti RK, et al. Best practice guide for the treatment of REM sleep behavior disorder (RBD). *J Clin Sleep Med* 2010; **6**(1): 85–95.

Further reading

Avidan AY, Kaplish N. The parasomnias: epidemiology, clinical features, and diagnostic approach. *Clin Chest Med* 2010; **31**(2): 353–70.

Kirsch DB. Diagnostic algorithm for parasomnias. In: Kushida C (ed) *Encyclopedia of Sleep Medicine*. New York: Academic Press, 2013. http://store. elsevier.com/Encyclopedia-of-Sleep/isbn-9780123786104/.

Lee-Chiong TL Jr. Parasomnias and other sleep-related movement disorders. *Prim Care* 2005; **32**(2): 415–34.

Malhotra RK, Avidan AY. Parasomnias and their mimics. *Neurol Clin* 2012; **30**(4): 1067–94.

Plante DT, Winkelman JW. Parasomnias. *Psychiatr Clin North Am* 2006; **29**(4): 969–87.

Tinuper P, Bisulli F, Provini F. The parasomnias: mechanisms and treatment. *Epilepsia* 2012; **53**(Suppl 7): 12–19.

12

Restless Legs Syndrome, Periodic Limb Movements, and Other Movement Disorders in Sleep

Raman Malhotra, MD

SLUCare Sleep Disorders Center and Department of Neurology and Psychiatry, Saint Louis University School of Medicine, USA

Introduction

Movements or behaviors can occur during sleep or around the time of sleep. These conditions may be pathological, leading to sleep disruption or injury, or may be benign and physiological. These movements or behaviors may be sporadic and intermittent, so diagnosis can be challenging to the clinician. Obtaining a detailed history from the patient or from a bed partner is key in distinguishing between different movements during sleep. Sleep-related movement disorders are simple, usually stereotyped movements that disturb sleep. Commonly included in this classification is restless legs syndrome which, though complex, is frequently associated with periodic limb movements of sleep which do fit this description. Complex motor behaviors of sleep, such as sleepwalking, confusional arousals, sleep terrors, and rapid eye movement (REM) sleep behavior disorder, are classified as parasomnias, and are also included in the differential diagnosis of abnormal movements during sleep. In addition to obtaining a detailed history regarding the movements, an attended, in-laboratory video polysomnogram may be helpful in diagnosis. This chapter will review sleep-related movement disorders.

Restless legs syndrome

Demographics

Restless legs syndrome (RLS) is a common disorder affecting up to 15% of the population.

Historically, epidemiological studies have been difficult to interpret due to the subjective nature of the symptoms and lack of standardized criteria, though this has improved with more recent international criteria for diagnosis. Recent population-based studies demonstrate that approximately 5% of the population report weekly symptoms, and 3% report moderate or severely distressing symptoms at least twice weekly. Most of these patients had not been appropriately diagnosed even though they had discussed their symptoms with their physicians.

Frequency of restless legs syndrome increases with age, with a prevalence of 2% between the ages of 8 and 18 and up to 19% in those over the age of 80. Women are more likely than men to suffer from restless legs syndrome, and their risk increases with parity. Northern European countries have a higher prevalence than Mediterranean populations. People of Asian or African descent seem to have a lower prevalence compared to Caucasians. Rates as low as 0.1% in Singapore to 0.9% in South Korea have been published.

Restless legs syndrome (primary) is hereditary in at least one-third of cases, possibly even higher. Family history is likely underestimated since many patients go undiagnosed with the condition. In some families inheritance is autosomal dominant, but there is more evidence that the genetic basis of this disorder is likely heterogeneous.

Sleep Medicine in Neurology, First Edition. Edited by Douglas B. Kirsch.
© 2014 John Wiley & Sons, Ltd. Published 2014 by John Wiley & Sons, Ltd.

Diagnosis and clinical presentation

Diagnostic criteria for the diagnosis of RLS in adults include an urge to move the legs, usually accompanied by uncomfortable or unpleasant sensations, the urge or unpleasant sensations begin or worsen during periods of rest or inactivity such as lying or sitting, the urge to move or unpleasant sensations are partially or totally relieved by movement, such as walking or stretching, and the urge to move or unpleasant sensations are worse in the evening or night. The condition must not be better explained by another sleep, medical disorder, medication or substance use (Box 12.1). Supportive clinical features include positive family history of the disorder, symptomatic response to dopaminergic therapy, and periodic limb movements of sleep or wakefulness as noted on polysomnogram.

The urge to move is often accompanied by an uncomfortable sensation, sometimes described as creeping, crawling, aching, pulling or prickly. The patient may find it very difficult to describe the sensation in detail. The symptoms are worse with inactivity and improved (temporarily) with movement such as walking, flexing, stretching, or

> ## Box 12.1 Diagnostic criteria for restless legs syndrome in adults
>
> - Patient reports urge to move the legs, usually accompanied or caused by uncomfortable and unpleasant sensations in the legs
> - The urge to move or the unpleasant sensations begin or worsen during periods of rest or inactivity
> - The urge to move or the unpleasant sensations are partially or totally relieved by movement
> - The urge to move or the unpleasant sensations are worse, or only occur, in the evening or night
> - The condition is not better explained by another current sleep disorder, medical or neurological disorder, mental disorder, medication use, or substance use disorder
>
> Reproduced from the *International Classification of Sleep Disorders: Diagnostic and Coding Manual*, 2nd edn.

tossing and turning in bed. In mild cases, the relief with movement may last for minutes whereas in severe cases, the symptoms may immediately return. Patients may rub or massage their legs, or apply warm or cold packs to their extremities to help relieve the discomfort. RLS may worsen during activities such as traveling by car or plane, or watching a show or movie. The symptoms can be apparent during the day but should be more pronounced at night. Peak symptoms are typically in the late evening or middle of the night, with the least amount of symptoms in the morning. The symptoms typically make it difficult for patients to fall asleep or stay asleep. The symptoms occur in the arms in up to half of patients, but typically start off in the lower extremities.

> ### ★ TIPS AND TRICKS
>
> A quick and easy way to remember the key clinical features of restless legs syndrome is to use the acronym URGE.
>
> U = urge or sensation to move the legs
> R = rest or stillness of the legs worsens the urge to move
> G = going is good (temporary relief with movement)
> E = evening or nighttime worsening of symptoms

Onset occurs at all ages from early childhood to late adulthood. Mean age of onset is difficult to determine due to delay in diagnosis. Symptoms typically progress over life, which contributes to this delay in diagnosis. Onset is at an earlier age in familial cases of RLS. Up to a third of RLS patients felt their symptoms started before the age of 10. Symptoms of RLS can fluctuate throughout a patient's lifetime though they seem to worsen with increasing age and during pregnancies in women.

In children, symptoms are sometimes misdiagnosed as "growing pains." Separate diagnostic criteria have been designed for children (ages 2–12) given the difficulties some may have in describing their symptoms. If children are able to meet all adult criteria above and relate a description in their own words regarding their leg discomfort, they meet criteria for RLS in the pediatric population. Another way for children to satisfy the criteria is meeting all four adult criteria and at least two of the following

Box 12.2 Medications that can worsen restless legs syndrome

Selective serotonin reuptake inhibitors
Norepinephrine reuptake inhibitors
Antihistamines
Sympathomimetics
Antipsychotics
Antiemetics

findings: sleep disturbance for age, biological parent or sibling with RLS, or a sleep study documenting periodic limb movement index of five or more movements per hour of sleep.

Physical and neurological exams are usually normal in patients with RLS. However, secondary RLS may be due to systemic or neurological disease. Decreased iron status is one major etiology of restless legs syndrome. Secondary RLS is also found in patients with uremia. As many as 50% of dialysis patients have RLS with some studies showing this leading to premature discontinuation of dialysis and association with increased morbidity and mortality. This high rate of RLS may be related to underlying anemia or neuropathy from the renal disease. Correction of renal function (including in cases of renal transplantation) has shown a resolution of RLS symptoms. RLS has also been shown to occur with pregnancy, spinal anesthesia, and use of certain medications (Box 12.2).

⚠ CAUTION

Medications that decrease levels of dopamine in the nervous system can lead to new or worsening RLS symptoms. This includes selective serotonin reuptake inhibitors (SSRI), tricyclic antidepressants, antiemetics, and many antipsychotics. Substances such as alcohol and caffeine have also been known to exacerbate RLS symptoms.

The most commonly reported neurological cause of secondary RLS is peripheral neuropathy. Up to 30% of pregnant patients develop RLS, usually in the last half of pregnancy. Symptoms stop soon after or immediately before delivery. Many other conditions have been associated with RLS, including migraines, chronic obstructive pulmonary disease,

Parkinson's disease, spinal cord lesions (demyelinating, neoplastic, infectious), multiple sclerosis, spinocerebellar atrophy and Charcot–Marie–Tooth type 2. RLS is seen more commonly in blood donors and in vegetarians who may not include enough iron in their diet.

Other causes of lower extremity discomfort need to be evaluated and excluded by history, examination, and sometimes additional testing. Arthritis, musculoskeletal pain, peripheral neuropathy, and peripheral vascular disease all need to be considered, though these conditions do not fit all essential criteria for restless legs syndrome. They may not improve with movement and may not worsen in the evening time. Patients with peripheral neuropathy will typically have symptoms distally in the feet, and may have decreased lower extremity reflexes and loss of sensation near the symptomatic area. Akathisia may also mimic RLS, though there is typically a history of use of neuroleptic use, absence of a circadian component, and more of a generalized description of an inner sense of restlessness as opposed to leg discomfort. Nocturnal leg cramps are also commonly misdiagnosed as restless legs syndrome. These are painful sensations in the legs associated with sudden muscle hardness or tightness occurring during the sleep period. They are relieved with forceful stretching of the muscle, releasing the muscle contraction.

Evaluation of restless legs syndrome sometimes includes testing such as nerve conduction studies to evaluate for peripheral neuropathy if there are suspicious findings on the neurological exam. Renal function tests and iron studies to look for secondary cause of RLS should also be performed. Iron deficiency cannot be ruled out by history or absence of anemia.

★ TIPS AND TRICKS

When evaluating iron status in patients with restless legs syndrome, it is important to look further than the normal reference range that most labs report for ferritin. Iron supplementation should be considered when a ferritin level is below 50 ng/mL. In addition, ferritin is an acute phase reactant and can be falsely elevated if the patient is suffering from an infection, such as an upper respiratory infection.

Overnight, attended polysomnography is not required for the diagnosis of restless legs syndrome, but can be helpful in specific clinical scenarios. Periodic limb movements of sleep are noted in 80% of patients with restless legs syndrome but are also noted at a high rate in the general population, making the finding often non-specific. Prevalence of periodic limb movements of sleep can range from 5% to 10% of the general population. Approximately 20% of patients found to have periodic limb movements of sleep on polysomnography had restless legs syndrome. As noted above, sleep studies can be helpful in pediatric diagnosis of restless legs syndrome by documenting presence of an elevated periodic limb movement index. Sleep studies are also helpful in evaluation for concurrent sleep-disordered breathing (sleep apnea) which can worsen symptoms of restless legs syndrome. Finally, in patients with persistent sleep complaints despite adequate treatment of restless legs syndrome, a sleep study may better characterize their sleep difficulties. Besides an elevated periodic limb movement index that is noted in approximately 80% of RLS patients, sleep studies in these patients demonstrate lower sleep efficiency and total sleep time, and an increased wake after sleep onset.

The suggested immobilization test (SIT) has been used to diagnose and assess the severity of restless legs syndrome. In this test, the patient remains in bed, reclined at 45°, with their legs stretched and eyes open. Surface electromyography (EMG) leads are placed on the right and left anterior tibialis muscles to quantify leg movements. Patients are told to try and remain still for the hour before their usual sleep period. They are also asked to subjectively grade their level of leg discomfort every 5 min. This test, primarily used in research studies, has been shown to have a sensitivity and specificity for restless legs syndrome of approximately 80%.

In-laboratory polysomnography to capture periodic limb movements of sleep can be time consuming and expensive, so alternative methods of detection have been attempted, including actigraphs (accelerometers) placed on the ankle or foot. This form of testing adds the advantage of capturing multiple nights of sleep in the patient's home environment. Several ratings scales have also been used to assess symptomatic response to medications. One of the more commonly used scales is the International Restless Legs Syndrome Study Group Rating Scale (IRLSS), which consists of 10 questions.

Pathophysiology

The underlying pathophysiology of restless legs syndrome is unclear, but most likely includes dopamine dysregulation. This disease may also involve impaired iron stores or regulation since iron serves as a co-factor for the production of dopamine. Both cerebrospinal fluid and advanced imaging studies of the central nervous system demonstrate low iron stores, particularly in the substantia nigra. Ultrasound and pathological specimens have shown reduced iron stores, but no evidence of degeneration or damage to dopaminergic cells. There may also be a component of decreased iron transport in the nervous system. True localization of the cause of restless legs syndrome has also been difficult as some studies suggest a peripheral nerve disorder while others assert spinal cord or brain pathology. Given the high positive family history noted in restless legs patients, genetics appears to play a key role in pathogenesis as well.

> **⚗ SCIENCE REVISITED**
>
> Iron is a necessary co-factor for the enzyme tyrosine hydroxylase, which is the rate-limiting step in the production of dopamine. Iron is also a component of the dopamine type 2 receptor, which may play a role in pathogenesis.

Management

Therapy for restless legs syndrome is individualized for each patient based upon severity and frequency of symptoms, along with other co-morbid medical conditions. Therapy is for symptomatic benefit and is not curative of the condition, so the benefit:risk ratio needs to be carefully considered before starting pharmacological therapy. Conservative treatments include avoiding medications and substances that can worsen restless legs syndrome. Warm baths, leg massage, relaxation techniques, cold packs, and good sleep hygiene may also help. Exercising or doing mentally stimulating activities before bed may also cause a modest improvement in some cases. Some studies have suggested that the use of compressive devices in the lower extremities for 1 hour per a day helped relieve some RLS symptoms at night.

It is also imperative that iron status be appropriately evaluated and corrected. Iron supplementation in patients with serum ferritin below 50 ng/mL has been shown to help symptoms of RLS, improve sleep, mood, and quality of life in RLS patients. Iron supplements can be given orally up to several times a day along with 100–200 mg vitamin C to help with absorption in both adults and children who are found to have a ferritin below 50 ng/mL. Intravenous iron has also been used in cases that have not responded to oral iron supplementation.

> ✋ CAUTION
>
> Oral iron can cause gastrointestinal symptoms such as abdominal discomfort and constipation.

In adults, the dopamine agonists ropinirole and pramipexole are FDA approved for restless legs syndrome and are considered first-line therapy by the most recent practice parameters from the American Academy of Sleep Medicine (AASM). These medications should be dosed 1–3 hours prior to symptom onset and titrated upwards until symptoms are controlled. Starting dose is 0.125 mg for pramipexole and 0.25 mg for ropinirole and both may need to be titrated upward depending on patient response. Sometimes, the medications will need to be dosed more than only at nighttime if symptoms occur during the day or evening. If breakthrough symptoms occur in between doses or in the middle of the night, there are different forms of dopamine agonists such as extended-release formulations and a transdermal option (rotigotine patch) that may be helpful. Ropinirole differs from pramipexole as it has a shorter half-life (6 hours) and is hepatically cleared. Pramipexole is renally cleared, and has a half-life of 8–10 hours. Dopamine agonists have caused development of impulse control disorders in patients using it to treat RLS, such as pathological gambling, sexual activity, or shopping. It is unclear when during treatment these behaviors may begin, but symptoms can occur months after initiating therapy.

> ✋ CAUTION
>
> Side-effects of dopamine agonists include sleepiness, sleep attacks, nausea, hallucinations, and compulsive behaviors.

Ergot-derived dopamine agonists, such as pergolide and cabergoline, have also been effective in treating restless legs syndrome. However, pergolide, despite its effectiveness, is not recommended for use in RLS due to its risk of heart valve damage. The same concern is present for carbergoline, though if other agents have failed, it can be cautiously considered.

In addition to the above side-effects, dopamine agonists can lead to augmentation. Augmentation is defined by earlier onset of symptoms during the day by at least 4 hours, or 2–4 hours earlier onset of symptoms and increased intensity of symptoms, spread to other parts of the body, or less relief with movement compared to before treatment. The increase in symptom severity cannot be accounted for by other factors (i.e. taking medications that worsen RLS) and there must have been a prior response to treatment. Augmentation may occur with both ropinirole or pramipexole at rates reported as high as 40% of patients and higher if carbidopa-levodopa is used. The mechanism behind augmentation is unknown, but well documented. If a patient suffers from augmentation, it is recommended that the dopamine agonist be discontinued and another agent initiated. Using a different dopaminergic agent can be helpful (i.e. switching from ropinirole to pramipexole), and experiencing augmentation from a certain medication does not necessarily mean that it cannot be used at some point in the future.

Levodopa (usually in the form of carbidopa-levodopa) has also been used in the treatment of restless legs syndrome. It is not recommended for long-term use mainly due to its short duration of action of 4–6 hours, and greater potential for augmentation compared to dopamine agonists. Levodopa may be a reasonable choice for patients with intermittent symptoms (less than three times a week) of a short duration. Side-effects are similar to those noted with the use of dopamine agonists.

Gabapentin is effective in the treatment of restless legs syndrome. It is commonly used when patients have a concomitant peripheral neuropathy since it is also helpful in relieving neuropathic pain. It is also used as treatment in children with restless legs syndrome after secondary causes (such as iron deficiency) have been evaluated and treated. Pregabalin is also effective in restless legs syndrome. Gabapentin enacarbil, which is a gamma-aminobutyric acid (GABA) analogue and prodrug to gabapentin, has increased absorption and sustained dose-dependent bioavailability, and is FDA approved for restless legs syndrome. Gabapentin and other related medications have not been associated with augmentation and are typically well tolerated.

Clonazepam is the best studied benzodiazepine in restless legs syndrome. Doses of 0.5–2 mg have been shown in some studies to be helpful in treating symptoms; the 2012 AASM practice parameters indicate that there is insufficient evidence to recommend it as monotherapy, and suggest its use as adjunct treatment. Other benzodiazepines such as diazepam, alprazolam, and temazepam have also been used to treat restless legs syndrome. Adverse effects of these medications include sedation and confusion. There does not seem to be a high risk of dose tolerance or abuse in the low doses used for restless legs syndrome. Though benzodiazepines seem to improve symptoms of restless legs syndrome, they do not seem to have a consistent effect on reducing the frequency of periodic limb movements of sleep.

Opioids were one of the earliest known treatments of restless legs syndrome. Due to the risk of abuse and addiction, this class of medications is typically only used if other agents have not been helpful. They can also be used when dopamine agents are withdrawn secondary to severe augmentation. Single bedtime doses of methadone, oxycodone, codeine, or tramadol are the opioids commonly used.

☝ CAUTION

Use of opioids in restless legs syndrome may lead to worsening of underlying sleep-disordered breathing, if present.

Other medications, such as clonidine and carbamazepine, have been effective in treatment of restless legs syndrome, though they have less evidence of their usefulness compared to the above medications.

In pregnancy, many of the above medications are not safe or may have unknown effects on the unborn child. Initially correcting iron status and implementing conservative measures (warm baths, leg massage, relaxation techniques) are recommended. In severe cases of restless legs syndrome during pregnancy, where the above recommendations are not helpful, opioids (FDA Pregnancy Category B) or benzodiazepines (Category D) may be considered.

Consequences

Patients with moderate-to-severe restless legs syndrome can experience significant decrease in their quality of life, similar to other chronic conditions such as osteoarthritis, diabetes, and depression. Quality of life measures such as vitality, physical functioning, and pain are markedly reduced in patients with RLS.

Periodic limb movement disorder

Periodic limb movements of sleep (PLMS) are episodes of repetitive, highly stereotyped limb movements that occur during sleep. They typically occur in the lower extremity and involve extension of the big toe, flexion of the ankle, knee, and hip. They can occur in both legs, unilaterally, or even alternate between legs. With polysomnography, a periodic limb movement index, or periodic limb movements per hour of sleep, is calculated. The limb movement must be 0.5–10 sec in duration as measured by surface EMG electrodes typically placed on the anterior tibialis muscle, or at times in the upper extremities if clinically indicated. The limb movement is only scored if it occurs in a series of at least four consecutive movements in intervals of 5–90 sec (Figure 12.1). PLMS usually appear in stage N1 and N2 sleep, and decrease in frequency in stage N3 and REM sleep. They may be associated with cortical arousals on electroencephalogram (EEG) or autonomic arousals (change in heart rate).

Periodic limb movements of sleep increase in incidence with increasing age, occurring in up to 34% of people over the age of 60. A periodic limb movement index above 5/hour is seen in up to 80% of restless legs syndrome patients, 70% of patients with REM sleep behavior disorder, and 65% of narcoleptics. Precipitation or aggravation of PLMS can occur with use of several medications such as serotonin reuptake inhibitor antidepressants, tricyclic antidepressants, and antipsychotics.

Periodic limb movement disorder (PLMD) is defined as a periodic limb movement of sleep index of greater than 15/hour (greater than 5/hour in children) and a clinical sleep disturbance or complaint of daytime fatigue. The condition should not be better

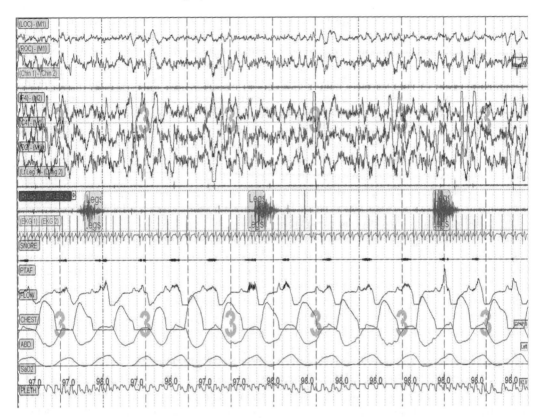

Figure 12.1 Channels are as follows: electrooculogram (left, LOC-M1; right, ROC-M1), chin electromyogram (Chin1-Chin2), electroencephalogram (right: frontal F4-M2, central C4-M1;occipital O2-M1), leg electromyography (Lt Leg 1 - Lt Leg 2, Rt Leg 1 - Rt Leg 2), electrocardiography (EKG1-EKG2), snore sensor (Snore), nasal pressure (PTAF), thermistor signal (FLOW), respiratory effort (CHEST, ABD), oxygen saturation (SAO2, PLETH). This 60-sec epoch of an overnight, attended sleep study shows three periodic leg movements in the right leg occurring during stage N3 sleep.

explained by another current sleep disorder, medical or neurological disorder, medication or substance use disorder. For example, a patient who already meets criteria for restless legs syndrome cannot also have periodic limb movement disorder. The patient may be conscious of the limb movements at night affecting their sleep, but typically their awareness of the frequency of disruption is not as evident as that noted on the sleep study. The bed partner or parent may help confirm abnormal movements during sleep. Besides sleep complaints, higher rates of depression, memory and attention difficulties, and oppositional behaviors have been reported in patients with periodic limb movement disorder.

There are limited studies on pharmacological treatment of periodic limb movement disorder, and in its most recent guidelines, the American Academy of Sleep Medicine made no specific evidence-based recommendations due to insufficient evidence. However, many of the studies looking at agents used to treat restless legs syndrome also measured the effects on periodic limb movement index on overnight sleep studies. Pramipexole, ropinirole, rotigotine, and gabapentin have all demonstrated significant reductions in periodic limb movement index on sleep studies. Other agents that have been used include clonazepam, melatonin, and valproate.

Other movement disorders of sleep

Sleep-related leg cramps

Sleep-related leg cramps are painful sensations in the leg or foot associated with sudden muscle hardness or tightness, indicating a strong muscle contraction. The calf or small muscles of the feet are the most commonly affected. The cramps can occur during sleep or the time around sleep, may appear during any sleep stage, and can cause insomnia or sleep disturbance. Forceful stretching of the affected muscle sometimes relieves the symptoms or releases the contraction. The cramp lasts seconds to several minutes and then usually spontaneously remits. There may be some tenderness and discomfort in the muscle for several hours after the cramp. This condition is very common, likely occurring at least once in the majority of people by the age of 50, increasing in frequency with age. Sleep-related leg cramps have been associated with diabetes mellitus, peripheral vascular disease, dehydration, metabolic and electrolyte disturbances, neuromuscular disease, and pregnancy. Stretching and exercise of the affected muscle may prevent or reduce occurrence. Quinine has been used in patients who have frequent episodes of leg cramps, but must be used with caution due to its severe side-effects, such as thrombocytopenia, and renal and liver disease. Verapamil and gabapentin have also been shown to reduce frequency of nocturnal leg cramps. Oral magnesium can be helpful in pregnant patients with sleep-related nocturnal leg cramps.

Rhythmic movement disorder

This disorder consists of repetitive, stereotyped, and rhythmic motor behaviors (not tremors) that involve large muscle groups and occur predominantly during drowsiness or sleep. The behaviors result in interference with normal sleep, significant impairment of daytime function, or self-inflicted bodily injury. If the movements do not result in any negative consequences (as stated above), they should not be considered a disorder. This disorder is typically seen in infants or children. There are several subtypes: body rocking, head banging, and head rolling. Body rocking may involve the entire body or may be limited to just the torso. Head banging involves forcibly lifting the head and repetitively banging it on the pillow, mattress, headboard or wall. Head rolling is side-to-side movements of the head with the child usually in the supine position. It is suggested that the movements act as a soothing effect before falling sleep, possibly via vestibular stimulation or self-stimulation. They typically occur during wake, stage N1, or N2 sleep. They can rarely occur in stage N3 or REM sleep.

The frequency of the movements is typically 0.5–2 per second. The duration is usually less than 15 min but may persist into light stages of sleep. Noise or disturbance can cause cessation of the activity, but typically the patient does not respond during the event. There is typically no recall of the event by the patient. The vast majority of children with sleep-related movements are otherwise normal. Up to 60% of infants may have these movements, body rocking being the most common. By 5 years of age, prevalence falls to 5%. It is rare to have this in adolescence or adulthood, though in adults with other central nervous system conditions, it is seen more commonly.

The rhythmic movements may lead to injury (especially head banging), and may also cause disruption to the sleep of other family members. Reassurance, ensuring a safe environment, and treating any underlying cause of awakenings at night (sleep apnea, restless legs) are the main treatments for this condition.

Sleep starts (hypnic jerks)

Sleep starts are sudden brief jerks at sleep onset, mainly in the arms and legs or involving the whole body. The jerks are associated with a feeling of falling, a sensory flash, auditory sound (bang), or hypnogogic dreams. The sensory symptoms may occur without the body jerk. The sleep starts are usually a single contraction that can be spontaneous or triggered by a stimulus. Excessive caffeine, emotional stress, and intense physical activity can increase the frequency of the events. Patients may not recall them occurring, and the motor activity may only be apparent to the bed partner or observer. Sleep starts are common with a prevalence of 70%. Only rarely, when they are frequent or intense, do they lead to insomnia. Though a polysomnogram is not required for diagnosis, sometimes it may be performed to rule out other motor disorders of sleep such as periodic limb movements or even seizures. On polysomnography, superficial limb EMG shows brief, high-amplitude potentials usually during drowsiness or stage N1 sleep. Management usually includes avoiding any known exacerbating factors and reassurance about the benign nature of the movements. In rare cases of insomnia related to sleep starts, benzodiazepines (usually clonazepam) have been used and may be effective.

Sleep-related bruxism

Sleep-related bruxism is grinding or clenching of the teeth during sleep. This occurs in a phasic or rhythmic pattern, or with sustained activity of the jaw muscles. The patient or an observer may notice the characteristic grinding sound. This disorder is associated with abnormal wear of the teeth, jaw discomfort, headache, or masseter muscle hypertrophy. Bruxism can also lead to sleep disruption, not only of the patient but also to their bed partner due to the noise. Bruxism may occur more with psychosocial stress and anxiety. It may also occur in relation to medication use or withdrawal or other medical conditions (Box 12.3). Bruxism can be intermittent, with patients being asymptomatic for several weeks between episodes, or it can occur nightly. This disorder is more common in childhood (14–17%) and then decreases with age, though up to a third continue to experience it in adulthood. There does seem to be a genetic component with 20–50% of patients having at least one family member with tooth grinding.

The diagnosis of sleep-related bruxism is based on history taking and an orofacial examination. An attended, in-laboratory polysomnogram may be indicated to demonstrate the disorder or exclude associated respiratory disturbances or parasomnias. Bruxism is suggested by a typical EMG artifact recorded on EEG derivations (Figure 12.2).

> **Box 12.3 Secondary causes of bruxism**
>
> Alcohol abuse
> Smoking
> Amphetamine use
> Medications: methylphenidate, antipsychotics, selective serotonin reuptake inhibitors, calcium channel blockers
> Parkinson's disease
> Tourette's syndrome
> Huntington's disease
> Sleep apnea
> Parasomnias
> Epilepsy
> Depression
> Dementia

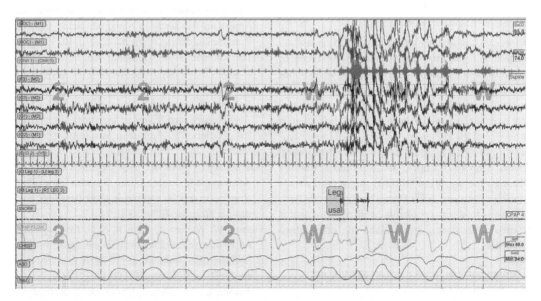

Figure 12.2 Channels are as follows: electrooculogram (left, LOC-M1; right, ROC-M1), chin electromyogram (Chin1-Chin3), electroencephalogram (left frontal F3-M2, left central C3-M2, left central C3-M2, left occipital O1-M2, right occipital O2-M2), electrocardiography (EKG2-V5), leg electromyography (Lt Leg 1 - Lt Leg 2, Rt Leg 1 - Rt Leg 2), CPAP flow (CPAP FLOW), respiratory effort (CHEST, ABD). This 60-sec epoch of an overnight, attended sleep study demonstrates bruxism. Repetitive muscle activity noted in the chin electromyography lead called rhythmic masticatory muscle activity is consistent with sleep-related bruxism.

Management of bruxism focuses on preventing damage to the teeth and other orofacial structures and reducing sensory or pain complaints. Damage prevention usually involves an occlusal appliance or bite splint along with clinical follow-up with a dentist. In stress-related bruxism, psychological intervention and counseling may be helpful. Rarely, medical treatments such as benzodiazepines or clonidine have been used for short-term management.

Propiospinal myoclonus at sleep onset

Propiospinal myoclonus at sleep onset is a rare spinal cord-mediated movement disorder consisting of sudden muscular jerks usually involving the abdominal and truncal muscles first, and then propagated to the limbs and neck. The jerks are of variable intensity and usually are flexor in nature. They occur during relaxed wakefulness and drowsiness, and typically disappear with mental activation or sleep onset. This condition has been described in acquired spinal cord lesions, restless legs syndrome, and paraneoplastic syndromes. Benzodiazepines and anticonvulsants have been reported to help reduce these movements.

Excessive fragmentary myoclonus

Excessive fragmentary myoclonus (EFM) is characterized by small movements of the fingers, toes, or corners of the mouth, or small muscle twitches resembling fasciculations that do not cause gross movement across a joint space. These movements are typically too small to be visible and the patient is unaware of the movements. Episodes of these myoclonic potentials typically last from 10 min to several hours. They often appear at sleep onset, continue through the non-REM (NREM) stages, and persist during REM sleep. It is unclear how often this finding leads to sleep complaints or disruption, as it is mostly seen during evaluations for other sleep disorders.

Hypnogogic foot tremor and alternating leg movement activation

Hypnogogic foot tremor (HFT) is a rhythmic movement of the feet or toes that occurs at the transition between wake and sleep or during light NREM sleep (stages N1 and N2). HFT is relatively common with a prevalence of at least 7.5% in patients having a sleep study performed for another reason. Patients move their feet or toes rhythmically for seconds to minutes. At times, there may be movement alternating between the two lower extremities (typically the anterior tibialis muscle) which is termed alternating leg muscle activation (ALMA). HFT is mostly reported in patients with other sleep disorders such as restless legs syndrome and sleep apnea. Many patients with ALMA are on antidepressant medications. In most patients, these movements do not interfere with sleep and may be found incidentally.

Further reading

Allen RP, Walters AS, Montplaisir J, et al. Restless legs syndrome prevalence and impact: REST general population study. *Arch Intern Med* 2005; **165**(11): 1286–92.

American Academy of Sleep Medicine. *International Classification of Sleep Disorders: Diagnostic and Coding Manual*, 2nd edn. Westchester, IL: American Academy of Sleep Medicine, 2005.

Aurora RN, Kristo DA, Bista SR, et al. The treatment of restless legs syndrome and periodic limb movement disorder in adults – an update for 2012: practice parameters with an evidence-based systematic review and meta-analysis: an American Academy of Sleep Medicine Clinical Practice Guideline. *Sleep* 2012;**35**(8): 1039–62.

Berry RB, Brooks R, Gamaldo CE, Harding SM, Marcus CL, Vaugh BV for the American Academy of Sleep Medicine. *The AASM Manual for the Scoring of Sleep and Associated Events: Rules, Terminology, and Technical Specifications, Version 2.0.* Darien, IL: American Academy of Sleep Medicine, 2012. www.aasmnet.org

Bliwise DL, Freeman A, Ingram CD, et al. Randomized, double-blind, placebo-controlled, short-term trial of ropinirole in restless legs syndrome. *Sleep Med* 2005; **6**(2): 141–7.

Hening W, Walters A, Allen R, et al. Impact, diagnosis, and treatment of restless legs syndrome in a primary care population: the REST primary care study. *Sleep Med* 2004; **5**: 237–46.

Kohyama J, Matsukura F, Kimura K, Tachibana N. Rhythmic movement disorder: polysomnographic study and summary of reported cases. *Brain Dev* 2002; **24**: 33–8.

Lavigne GJ, Khoury S, Abe S, Yamaguchi T, Raphael K. Bruxism physiology and pathology: an overview for clinicians. *J Oral Rehabil* 2008; **35**(7): 476–94.

Montplaisir J, Lapierre O, Warnes H, Pelletier G. The treatment of the restless legs syndrome with or without periodic leg movements in sleep. *Sleep* 1992; **15**(5): 391–5.

Rye DB, Trotti LM. Restless legs syndrome and periodic leg movements of sleep. *Neurol Clin* 2012; **30**(4): 1137–66.

Walters AS. Clinical identification of the simple sleep-related movement disorders. *Chest* 2007; **131**(4): 1260–6.

Winkelman JW, Johnston L. Augmentation and tolerance with long-term pramipexole treatment of restless legs syndrome (RLS). *Sleep Med* 2004; **5**(1): 9–14.

Winkelman JW, Sethi KD, Kushida CA, et al. Efficacy and safety of pramipexole in restless legs syndrome. *Neurology* 2006; **67**(6): 1034–9.

Sleep and Neurological Disorders

Maryann C. Deak, MD

Harvard Medical School, Brigham and Women's Hospital, USA

Introduction

Sleep disorders are common in patients with neurological disease involving either the central or peripheral nervous system. Recognizing and treating sleep disorders is an important aspect of managing patients with neurological problems. The relationship between sleep and neurological disorders is often bidirectional, with the potential for each disorder to affect the disease course and outcome of the other. The underlying cause of sleep problems is complex and multifactorial in neurological patients (Box 13.1).

Parkinson's disease and other alpha-synucleinopathies

Sleep disorders are common in Parkinson's disease (PD) and in other disorders associated with parkinsonism that share a common pathophysiology (i.e.

Box 13.1 Contributors to sleep disruption in neurological disorders

Damage to sleep-regulating centers of the brain and brainstem
Medication side-effects
Motor symptoms
Pain
Autonomic dysfunction
Seizures or other episodic neurological events
Psychiatric disorders such as depression and anxiety
Primary sleep disorders such as obstructive sleep apnea

alpha-synuclein deposits), including Lewy body dementia (LBD) and multiple system atrophy (MSA). PD is a progressive, neurodegenerative disorder characterized by resting tremor, bradykinesia (i.e. slowness of movement), rigidity, and postural instability. PD is the second most common neurodegenerative disorder after Alzheimer's dementia, affecting 1–2% of the population over age 65 and increasing in prevalence with age. Abnormal sleep is present in approximately 50% of patients with PD. In fact, sleep problems, particularly rapid eye movement (REM) sleep behavior disorder (RBD) and excessive daytime sleepiness, are often present early in PD prior to the manifestation of motor symptoms.

Rapid eye movement sleep behavior disorder, hypersomnia, and insomnia are the most frequently encountered sleep problems in PD, with RBD being the most common. As a neurodegenerative process, PD directly affects the thalamocortical arousal system, as well as sleep-regulating centers in the brainstem. Other contributing factors include motor and autonomic symptoms, dopaminergic medication side-effects, co-morbid sleep disorders such as obstructive sleep apnea and restless legs syndrome, and co-morbid mood disorders.

Lewy body dementia and MSA are examples of other synucleinopathies. Alpha-synuclein is a protein that abnormally accumulates in Lewy bodies in both PD and LBD and in oligodendrocyte inclusions in MSA. LBD is the second most common cause of dementia after AD. It is characterized by cognitive impairment, parkinsonism, and hallucinations. MSA is an uncommon disorder characterized by autonomic failure associated with either

Sleep Medicine in Neurology, First Edition. Edited by Douglas B. Kirsch.
© 2014 John Wiley & Sons, Ltd. Published 2014 by John Wiley & Sons, Ltd.

parkinsonism or cerebellar ataxia. As in PD, sleep disorders are common in both LBD and MSA.

REM sleep behavior disorder

Rapid eye movement sleep behavior disorder is characterized by loss of muscle atonia during REM sleep, which is accompanied by enactment of often violent dreams (Figure 13.1). The movements in RBD appear purposeful, are not stereotyped, and are performed with eyes closed. There is significant risk of injury to the patient or the bed partner in RBD. A diagnosis of RBD is based on the presence of REM sleep without atonia on polysomnography, in conjunction with a history or polysomnographic documentation of dream enactment behavior (see Figure 13.1).

Rapid eye movement sleep behavior disorder is present in 15–60% of patients with PD, with rates approaching 90% in LBD and MSA. RBD often precedes the development of the associated alpha-synucleinopathy by an average of 10 years, although intervals of up to 50 years have been described. Studies have shown that 40% of RBD patients develop parkinsonism and/or dementia within approximately a decade after the onset of RBD symptoms, while 65% develop it after two decades. The presumed pathophysiology of RBD is related to damage to the brainstem nuclei controlling atonia during REM sleep, most likely the subcoeruleus nucleus in the pons.

Management of RBD involves securing the sleeping environment to avoid injury to the patient and the bed partner. Examples of suggested measures include sleeping on a mattress on the floor, padding corners of furniture, and removal of sharp objects or other potentially dangerous objects from the bedroom. Patients and bed partners may consider sleeping in separate rooms until symptoms are well controlled. With regard to pharmacological management, there are no large placebo-controlled trials to guide treatment decisions for RBD. However, recent published best practice guidelines indicate that clonazepam, at a nightly dose of 0.25–2.0 mg, and melatonin, at a nightly dose of 3–12 mg, are likely the most effective pharmacological options. To limit risk of side-effects, the lowest effective dose should be used. Potential side-effects of clonazepam

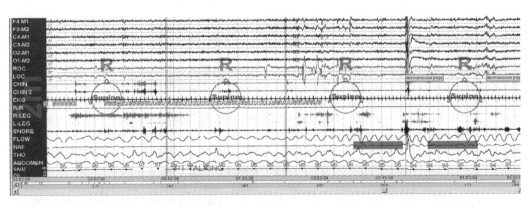

Figure 13.1 30-sec REM epoch from polysomnography of a patient with RBD. Evidence of lack of muscle atonia is present in chin and limb leads. The technician noted that the patient was talking during REM sleep.

include morning sedation, confusion, and motor incoordination. As a result, patients on this medication should be monitored closely, particularly older or neurologically impaired patients. Potential side-effects of melatonin include morning sedation or headaches, although side-effects are generally infrequent.

Hypersomnia

Excessive daytime sleepiness (EDS) is common in PD, occurring in approximately one-third of patients. Hypersomnia is often multifactorial, related to areas of the brain affected by the disease process itself, sleep disruption by motor symptoms or non-motor symptoms such as nocturia, co-morbid sleep disorders such as RBD and sleep-disordered breathing, as well as medication side-effects.

Between 1% and 4% of PD patients experience sleep attacks, which are defined as episodes of sudden onset of sleep without warning. Most concerning is the occurrence of sleep attacks during driving, and patients with sleep attacks should be warned not to drive. Sleep attacks are strongly associated with therapy with dopamine agonists. The risk of sleep attacks also appears to be greater in older patients, those with longer disease durations, and possibly greater in men compared to women.

> ⚠ **CAUTION**
>
> Sleep attacks can occur in up to 4% of patients with PD and carry significant risk for injury.

A careful history and physical examination should be performed in PD patients to determine potential underlying cause of EDS. Possible secondary contributing factors such as co-morbid sleep disorders or medications should be identified in these patients and addressed whenever possible. Appropriate sleep hygiene should also be stressed. There are few studies available to guide treatment of sleepiness in PD, and there are no FDA-approved medications for the treatment of EDS in patients with PD. The wake-promoting agent modafinil has been studied in PD and was well tolerated. However, studies examining efficacy of modafinil for treatment of EDS in PD have yielded mixed results, suggesting that modafinil improves subjective perception of wakefulness, but does not improve objective measures of alertness. Use of this medication for treatment of EDS in PD remains controversial.

Insomnia

Both sleep onset and sleep maintenance insomnia have been described in patients with PD but sleep maintenance insomnia is more common. Approximately 40% of patients with PD and 50% of patients with MSA complain of sleep fragmentation. LBD is also commonly associated with sleep disturbance, and sleep disturbance in LBD is more common than in Alzheimer's dementia.

Insomnia may be related to core motor symptoms of PD, non-motor symptoms such as nocturia, symptoms of anxiety and depression, co-morbid sleep disorders such as sleep-disordered breathing or restless legs syndrome, and medication side-effects. Similarly, sleep problems in MSA correlate with longer disease duration, more severe motor symptoms, depression, and length of treatment with dopaminergic medications.

With regard to treatment of insomnia symptoms in PD, maximization of control of motor and non-motor symptoms of PD can be beneficial. Co-morbid sleep and psychiatric disorders should be addressed. Sleep hygiene, including improving the sleeping environment and maintaining a regular sleep schedule, should also be stressed. Few studies have examined the efficacy of sedative-hypnotic medication in PD and there are insufficient data to make specific recommendations. Melatonin may improve subjective perception of sleep quality, but it is unclear if sleep quality objectively improves.

Sleep-disordered breathing

Sleep-disordered breathing, including nocturnal stridor and obstructive sleep apnea, is common in MSA. Of particular concern is the possibility of nocturnal stridor, which is potentially life threatening. Stridor results from partial obstruction of the larynx, and it is associated with a high-pitched noise. Between 20% and 40% of MSA patients experience nocturnal stridor. Stridor can often be effectively treated with continuous positive airway pressure.

> ⚠ **CAUTION**
>
> Nocturnal stridor, which is present in 20–40% of patients with MSA, is potentially life threatening.

Obstructive sleep apnea has not been shown to be more common in PD compared with age-matched controls. However, as a common cause of sleep disturbance and EDS in the general population, patients with PD and sleep problems should be screened for OSA.

Alzheimer's disease and other dementias

Alzheimer's disease (AD) and other dementias are frequently associated with sleep disruption. AD is the most common form of dementia, affecting 60–80% of demented patients. LBD (discussed above) accounts for approximately 15–25% of dementia cases. Other causes of dementia include frontotemporal dementias and progressive supranuclear palsy, as well as vascular dementia. However, most of the literature on sleep disturbance in dementia involves patients with AD.

Alzheimer's disease is defined by progressive memory impairment, associated with impairment in one or more other domains such as apraxia, aphasia or executive function that affects daytime functioning. Approximately 25–50% of patients with AD experience sleep disruption. Sleep disturbance is a significant factor contributing to institutionalization of patients with AD and other dementias. Sleep disturbance in AD often consists of insomnia, circadian rhythm disturbance, nocturnal agitation, and nocturnal wandering. The cause of sleep disturbance is often multifactorial in dementia patients.

Insomnia and circadian rhythm disturbance

Insomnia in dementia may manifest as difficulty initiating sleep, nocturnal or early morning awakenings, and/or episodes of nocturnal agitation or confusion. Insomnia in AD is attributable to a combination of factors. AD directly affects the suprachiasmatic nucleus and other areas of the brain important for sleep regulation and circadian rhythms. Many patients develop an irregular sleep-wake rhythm, likely related to disease progression. Daytime sleep has been shown to increase with disease severity. Other potential contributors to insomnia and circadian disturbance are medication side-effects, psychiatric disorders such as anxiety, co-morbid sleep disorders such as obstructive sleep apnea, and poor sleep hygiene. Poor sleep hygiene may include spending excessive amounts of time in bed, reduced daytime physical activity, and limited daytime light exposure.

> ★ **TIPS AND TRICKS**
>
> Insomnia can present in a variety of ways in AD, including difficulty initiating sleep, difficulty maintaining sleep, and/or episodes of nocturnal agitation or confusion.

Treatment of insomnia in AD requires first a detailed history and physical examination to determine possible contributing factors. Co-morbid disorders should be addressed. Studies have examined behavioral and pharmacological methods of treating sleep disturbance in AD.

Behavioral intervention is likely more effective than pharmacological treatment and carries a low risk of adverse events (Box 13.2). Bright light therapy in the morning or all day consisting of light intensity greater than 2500 lux may reduce nighttime sleep fragmentation, increase the night sleep period, and reduce daytime sleepiness. Other behavioral interventions such as increasing daytime physical activity, decreasing time spent in bed during the day, and creating a structured bedtime routine have also demonstrated promising results for improving sleep quality.

> ★ **TIPS AND TRICKS**
>
> Behavioral intervention for treatment of insomnia in AD is likely more effective than pharmacological management and carries a low risk of adverse events.

With regard to pharmacological management, evidence to guide treatment is limited. Use of melatonin for insomnia has lead to mixed results, with several studies showing no benefit. Melatonin may have some potential benefit when combined

> **Box 13.2 Behavioral intervention for treatment of sleep disturbance in AD**
>
> Light therapy
> Increasing daytime physical activity
> Decreasing time spent in bed during the day
> Structured bedtime routine
> Decreasing nighttime noise and light

with bright light therapy, but further studies are warranted in this area. Acetylcholinesterase inhibitors, which are often used in the treatment of AD, may improve some aspects of sleep architecture such as REM density, but the impact on sleep is limited. Additionally, donepezil, galantamine, and memantine may cause insomnia as a side-effect. Sedative-hypnotic medications, including benzodiazepines and non-benzodiazepines, have not been extensively studied for treatment of insomnia in dementia and carry the risk of sedation and confusion.

Obstructive sleep apnea

Obstructive sleep apnea (OSA) is more common in AD compared to the general population. Interestingly, there is a possible association between the apolipoprotein E ε4 allele, which increases the risk of AD, and OSA. OSA has the potential to cause or worsen cognitive impairment. A recent study demonstrated that obstructive sleep apnea is associated with a significantly higher likelihood of developing cognitive impairment or dementia over 5 years of follow-up, with the risk increasing with more sleep apnea events or a lower oxygen nadir. A preliminary study demonstrated that positive airway pressure, which is the treatment of choice for OSA, may slow cognitive decline and improve mood, sleep quality, and daytime sleepiness in patients with AD.

REM sleep behavior disorder

Rapid eye movement sleep behavior disorder, which is discussed above, has also been described in AD, progressive supranuclear palsy, and other types of dementia. However, the RBD is significantly less common in these disorders compared to alpha-synucleinopathies.

Epilepsy

Epilepsy is defined as the occurrence of recurrent unprovoked seizures. Seizures are characterized by abnormal electrical activity in the brain resulting in undesirable behavior or sensation. About 20% of patients with epilepsy experience seizures principally at night, which have the potential to disrupt sleep (Figure 13.2). Sleep complaints are common in epilepsy, as are sleep disorders such as obstructive sleep apnea.

Overview of sleep disruption in epilepsy

Patients with epilepsy are twice as likely to report sleep disturbance compared to healthy controls. Sleep disturbance can result in daytime sleepiness, reduced quality of life, and impairment of daytime functioning, including cognitive functioning. Poor sleep quality or sleep deprivation also has the potential to increase seizure frequency.

Seizures can adversely affect sleep, while sleep disturbances can worsen seizure control; the cause of sleep disturbance is complex in epilepsy patients. Both interictal discharges and seizures can be activated by sleep. Nocturnal seizures and antiepileptic drugs (AEDs) alike can affect sleep quality. Seizures result in reduced REM sleep and increased sleep fragmentation. Treatment of seizures with AEDs may improve sleep. However, AEDs can also negatively affect sleep architecture and daytime alertness. For example, phenytoin likely decreases sleep efficiency and REM sleep, while carbamazepine decreases REM sleep. Newer AEDs such as lamotrigine or levetiracetam are less likely to affect sleep architecture. In addition, some antiepileptic medications such as barbiturates have the potential to worsen co-morbid sleep disorders like OSA. Co-morbid sleep disorders such as OSA and co-morbid psychiatric disorders such as anxiety and depression also adversely affect sleep quality in epilepsy patients.

Evaluation of sleep complaints and/or daytime sleepiness in epilepsy patients requires careful consideration of possible contributing factors, including a detailed history of seizure control as well as possible co-morbid disorders. Control of seizures should be maximized if this is a contributing factor. The patient's AED regimen should be examined and possible adverse effects should be considered. Evaluation and treatment of co-morbid sleep disorders such as OSA are essential. Finally, treatment of mood disorders is an important aspect of managing sleep complaints.

Obstructive sleep apnea

Obstructive sleep apnea is common in epilepsy, with recent reports indicating a prevalence of 10% in unselected adults with epilepsy, although rates may be higher (up to 30%) in patients with refractory epilepsy. One study found that children with epilepsy and sleep complaints had a 20% prevalence of OSA.

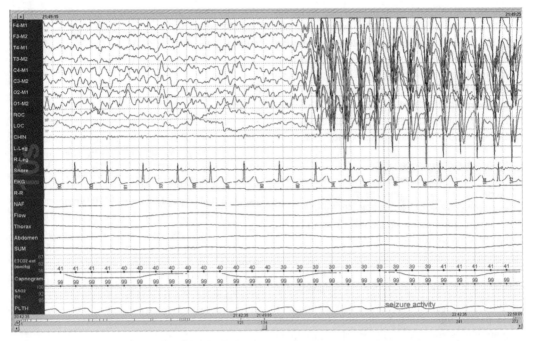

Figure 13.2 This is a 10-sec epoch of a polysomnogram (Nihon Kohden, Foothills Ranch, CA). The top eight leads are EEG leads, followed by two ocular leads (ROC/LOC), chin EMG (CHIN), leg EMG (L-LEG, R-LEG), snore channel, EKG with R-R interval, nasal pressure signal (NAF), oronasal thermistor (Flow), respiratory effort bands (Thorax and Abdomen) with a SUM channel, end-tidal carbon dioxide (ETCO2) with capnogram, oxygen saturation (SaO2), and plethysmography signal (PLTH). This image demonstrates the onset of a spike-wave complex just after the halfway point of the epoch; the spike-waves appear generalized and occur at 3 Hz frequency.

Risk factors for OSA in epilepsy patients include male sex, older age, and obesity. Both epilepsy and epilepsy treatment contribute to the increased prevalence of OSA. Some AEDs may increase the risk of OSA either through direct impact on the upper airway and arousal mechanisms or by causing weight gain. Vagus nerve stimulators have the potential to worsen obstructive sleep apnea. There is evidence that seizures themselves may exacerbate obstructive sleep apnea.

> ☆ **TIPS AND TRICKS**
>
> Treatment of obstructive sleep apnea with continuous positive airway pressure (CPAP) in epilepsy patients has the potential to improve seizure control.

Obstructive sleep apnea likely increases seizure frequency in epilepsy patients. Additionally, it has the potential to worsen daytime functioning, quality of life, cognition, and mood disorders. Several studies have suggested that treatment with CPAP improves seizure control. Treatment of OSA results in improved seizure control in approximately one-third of patients with co-morbid epilepsy and OSA. A recent retrospective study found that epilepsy patients on stable AED regimens who are compliant with CPAP have better seizure control compared to patients who are non-compliant.

Seizures versus parasomnias

Consideration of the interplay between epilepsy and sleep would not be complete without a discussion of epilepsy and parasomnias. In particular, nocturnal frontal lobe epilepsy (NFLE) is often difficult to distinguish from parasomnias due to the similarities between seizure semiology and clinical manifestations of non-REM parasomnias. Frontal lobe seizures generally consist of posturing, vocalization, motor activity such as pelvic thrusting or bicycling, and occasionally walking or running. NFLE events generally arise out of stage 2 sleep. Non-REM parasomnias, which generally arise out of slow-wave sleep, can consist of vocalization, ambulation, and semi-purposeful behaviors. Video-electroencephalography (EEG) is generally needed to make a diagnosis. However, certain key clinical features can help make a distinction between non-REM parasomnias and NFLE.

> ★ TIPS AND TRICKS
>
> A detailed history, in conjunction with overnight video EEG, can help to distinguish between nocturnal frontal lobe seizures and non-REM parasomnias.

Seizures consistent of stereotypical behavior, i.e. specific behaviors are repeated with every episode, while parasomnias are typically not stereotyped. Patients with seizures generally experience multiple events per night (often three or more), whereas parasomnias do not occur more than once or twice during a night. During non-REM parasomnias, patients often engage in complex, semi-purposeful, directed activities that involve interacting with objects or people in the environment. This type of behavior is not typical for NFLE. Recall for non-REM parasomnias is much less common compared to frontal lobe seizures. Non-REM parasomnias are more likely to begin in childhood, whereas NFLE can begin at any age. Additionally, other historical clues such as a family history of seizures or daytime epileptic events can be helpful in making a distinction. Because epilepsy and non-REM parasomnias are treated differently, response or lack of response to treatment can also be helpful in clarifying a diagnosis. NFLE is treated with AEDs appropriate for focal epilepsies. Treatment of non-REM parasomnias includes precautions for environmental safety, optimizing sleep hygiene, treating co-morbid sleep disorders, and occasionally use of medication such as benzodiazepines.

Stroke

Stroke is an acute focal neurological deficit caused by a vascular event. Stroke is one of the most common neurological disorders, with incidence estimates of 2–3 per 1000 per year. Stroke and sleep disorders have an important bidirectional relationship. Sleep disorders modify vascular risk factors and increase the risk of stroke. Stroke can cause or worsen underlying sleep disorders.

Sleep-disordered breathing

Approximately 50–70% of acute stroke patients have sleep-disordered breathing, either OSA or central sleep apnea (CSA). OSA is more common than CSA. Sleep-disordered breathing severity often improves in the 3–6 months following stroke, although prevalence rates of sleep-disordered breathing, defined by an Apnea Hypopnea Index (AHI) greater than 10, remain high. CSA is more likely to improve following stroke. OSA is associated with a number of potential adverse consequences, including increased risk of stroke, as well as affecting outcomes after stroke. The impact of CSA is less clear, and CSA may be a consequence of stroke rather than a clear contributor to increased stroke risk.

> ★ TIPS AND TRICKS
>
> Stroke patients should be screened for sleep-disordered breathing due to high prevalence estimates and potential for increased morbidity and mortality.

A number of prospective cohort or cross-sectional cohort studies have demonstrated an increased risk of stroke in OSA patients with odds or hazard ratios ranging between 1.6 and 3.8. Increased severity of OSA, as evidenced by higher AHI, is associated with greater stroke risk. Proposed mechanisms for the association between OSA and stroke include OSA-induced sympathetic activation, hypertension, hypoxemia, changes in cerebral blood flow, increased risk of cardiac arrhythmias, as well as atherosclerosis. OSA is also associated with other vascular risk factors such as diabetes mellitus and obesity.

Obstructive sleep apnea has also been shown to affect clinical course following stroke (Box 13.3). Sleep-disordered breathing is associated with less favorable neurological short- and long-term outcomes, including worse functional outcome, longer hospitalization, and increased mortality. Severe sleep apnea is associated with a higher risk of recurrent stroke.

Box 13.3 Potential consequences of obstructive sleep apnea in stroke patients

Less favorable functional neurological
   outcome
Longer hospitalization
Increased risk of recurrent stroke
Increased risk of cardiac complications such as
   arrhythmias
Increased mortality

Continuous positive airway pressure remains the treatment of choice for OSA. CPAP has been shown to improve sleep quality and daytime sleepiness, and reduce blood pressure and other cardiovascular risk factors. There is a paucity of randomized controlled clinical trials examining treatment with CPAP in stroke patients. The available data suggest that stroke patients on CPAP long term likely have a reduced risk or a delayed recurrence of vascular events after stroke. One study examining patients with OSA after stroke who were adherent with CPAP therapy versus those who were not adherent suggests that treatment with CPAP reduces risk of mortality from cardiovascular events including stroke. Commonly cited obstacles to CPAP adherence in stroke patients include neurological impairment, mask discomfort, and claustrophobia. While additional randomized controlled studies are needed, CPAP is currently recommended for potential primary and secondary stroke prevention. CSA is often treated with CPAP, oxygen or adaptive servo-ventilation.

Other sleep-wake disturbances

Other sleep-wake disturbances (SWD) common in stroke patients include insomnia, increased need for sleep, and excessive daytime sleepiness. SWD is most common in the acute phase following stroke and may improve in the months following stroke. The underlying cause of SWD following stroke is related to the brain damage caused by the stroke, environmental factors, mood symptoms, co-morbid medical conditions such as cardiac failure, sleep-disordered breathing, pain, medications, and other possible post-stroke complications such as urinary or respiratory infections. Sleep-related movement disorders such as restless legs syndrome may also occur *de novo* following stroke and contribute to disturbed sleep. There are few data to guide management of SWD in stroke patients. Co-morbid medical, psychiatric and sleep disorders should be addressed, when possible, and environmental conditions should be optimized.

Multiple sclerosis

Multiple sclerosis (MS) is characterized by T cell-mediated demyelination of focal areas of the brain and spinal cord, resulting in neurological deficits. MS is a leading cause of disability in young adults, affecting over 1 million people worldwide. MS is at least twice as common in women as men. Approximately 50% of patients with MS report sleep-related problems. Moreover, sleep disorders are often underrecognized in the MS population.

Insomnia

Approximately 40% of MS patients report difficulty initiating or maintaining sleep. The causes of insomnia symptoms in MS are varied. Pain is a common symptom in MS with the potential to disturb sleep. Common causes of pain in MS include neuropathic pain or pain related to muscle spasms. Nocturia or urinary incontinence, which affects up to 80% of patients with MS, also causes sleep fragmentation. Medications commonly used in the treatment of MS, including interferon and corticosteroids, may cause or worsen insomnia. Finally, co-morbid psychiatric or sleep disorders are common in MS. Major depressive disorder is present in an estimated 25% of MS patients. Other primary sleep disorders such as nocturnal movement disorders or sleep-disordered breathing may also cause difficulty initiating or maintaining sleep and non-restorative sleep in MS.

Treatment of insomnia in MS must include a thorough investigation for possible contributing factors. Targeting underlying causes such as pain, urinary symptoms, or co-morbid conditions should be the first line of treatment. Non-pharmacological treatment for insomnia, such as cognitive behavioral therapy, and pharmacological treatments can be considered, although there are few data available to guide treatment of primary insomnia in MS patients.

Restless legs syndrome

Restless legs syndrome (RLS) is more prevalent in MS compared to the general population. A recent study showed that women with MS were almost three times more likely to have RLS than women without RLS, and four times more likely to have severe RLS. The increased prevalence of RLS in MS may be related to a pathophysiological link between the two disorders. One study showed that MS patients with RLS had more cervical cord lesions on magnetic resonance spectroscopy compared to those without RLS, suggesting that the occurrence of RLS may be related to cervical cord damage.

Because MS is commonly associated with sensory symptoms such as dysesthesias and paresthesias, it is important to distinguish RLS from sensory symptoms associated with MS. All four diagnostic criteria must be present to make a diagnosis of RLS, including an urge to move the legs, often accompanied by unpleasant sensations; initiating or worsening of symptoms at rest; partial or total relief of symptoms with movement; and worsening of symptoms in the evening or night compared to the day. Treatment of RLS in MS is similar to treatment in patients without MS, with dopaminergic agents or anticonvulsants such as gabapentin being the mainstays of treatment. Patients with MS should also be screened for other possible secondary causes of RLS such as iron deficiency.

> ## ⚠ CAUTION
>
> A careful history is required to distinguish between MS-associated sensory symptoms and RLS.

Sleep-disordered breathing

Both central and obstructive sleep apnea have been described in MS patients. However, the prevalence of sleep-disordered breathing (SDB) in MS is unclear due to a lack of large-scale epidemiological studies. The incidence of SDB in MS is likely similar to the general population. Treatment of SDB in MS is also similar to the general population, with CPAP being the treatment of choice.

Narcolepsy

While there are no studies in MS patients examining the prevalence of narcolepsy, MS is thought to be a possible symptomatic cause of narcolepsy. Both disorders are linked to similar human leukocyte antigen expression, suggesting a possible common autoimmune pathology. There are no clear guidelines for treatment of narcolepsy in MS, and treatment options are similar to the general population. Modafinil is a mainstay of narcolepsy treatment, and may also be effective in MS-related chronic fatigue.

Neuromuscular disease

Neuromuscular disease includes a range of disorders of the motor unit, including disorders that affect brainstem motor neurons, anterior horn cells in the spinal cord, motor roots, peripheral nerves, neuromuscular junctions, and muscles. Sleep disorders are common in neuromuscular diseases. Due to the presence of motor weakness, SDB, including OSA, central sleep apnea, and nocturnal alveolar hypoventilation, is the most common sleep problem in patients with neuromuscular disease. Patients with neuromuscular disease may also experience sleep disturbance due to pain, abnormal movements or spasticity, co-morbid psychiatric disorders or medication side-effects. Hypersomnia may also occur in patients with neuromuscular disease, particularly myotonic dystrophy.

> ## ★ TIPS AND TRICKS
>
> Sleep-disordered breathing is the most common sleep problem in patients with neuromuscular disease.

Sleep-disordered breathing

Patients with neuromuscular disease should be screened for SDB, due to high prevalence and potential impact on quality of life and survival. Neuromuscular diseases commonly associated with SDB include amyotrophic lateral sclerosis (motor neuron disease), myasthenia gravis (neuromuscular junction disease), acute inflammatory demyelinating polyradiculoneuropathy (peripheral nerve disease), and muscular dystrophies (muscle disease) including myotonic dystrophies. Patients with neuromuscular disease develop SDB primarily due to upper airway muscle weakness resulting in increased resistance and OSA, as well as chest wall and diaphragmatic weakness resulting in alveolar hypoventilation and restrictive lung disease. A combination of OSA and alveolar hypoventilation, and possibly CSA, is common in this patient population. Work-up for suspected SDB should include overnight polysomnography, including end-tidal PCO_2. Arterial blood gas and pulmonary function testing is also important in patients with suspected hypoventilation.

Sleep-disordered breathing should be identified and treated due to the potential negative impact on quality of life, as well as increased morbidity and mortality. While more studies are needed to identify the impact of treatment in patients with neuromuscular disease, treatment likely improves daytime symptoms and quality of life. Treatment with non-invasive positive pressure ventilation increases survival in amyotrophic lateral sclerosis. Positive airway pressure in the form of CPAP or bilevel PAP is the treatment of choice for SDB in neuromuscular disease. Bilevel PAP is often required due to the high prevalence of alveolar hypoventilation. Supplemental oxygen may be added in some cases, although American Academy of Sleep Medicine guidelines recommend addition of oxygen only in patients with low awake oxygen saturation or when oxygen saturation remains low during sleep despite optimization of pressure support and respiratory rate with non-invasive positive pressure ventilation.

☆ TIPS AND TRICKS

Treatment of SDB can improve survival in neuromusclar disease, particularly motor neuron disease.

Hypersomnia

Central hypersomnia has been described in patients with myotonic dystrophy type 1 (DM 1), an autosomal dominant disorder that is the most common adult-onset muscular dystrophy. Approximately 70–80% of patients with DM 1 complain of excessive daytime sleepiness. While SDB is common in DM 1, daytime sleepiness may persist despite adequate treatment of SDB. In addition, sleepiness appears to occur independently of polysomnographic abnormalities in DM 1. Evidence suggests that hypersomnia in DM 1 is likely caused by dysfunction of sleep regulation caused by damage in the brain and brainstem. Treatment of central hypersomnia in DM 1 consists first of identifying and treating possible contributors such as SDB. There may be a role for

use of stimulant medications, such as methylphenidate or modafinil, to treat hypersomnia. However, studies to date exploring use of stimulant medications in DM 1 have yielded mixed results, and more research is needed in this area.

Conclusion

Sleep disorders are common in neurological disease. The underlying cause of sleep complaints is often complex in neurological patients. Both the neurological disease process and treatment of neurological disease may contribute to sleep disturbance. Sleep disorders may increase the risk of neurological disorders or worsen symptoms. An important future area of study is the appropriate treatment of sleep disorders in neurological disease.

Further reading

Aurora RN, Zak R, Maganti R, et al. Best practice guide for the treatment of REM sleep behavior disorder (RBD). *J Clin Sleep Med* 2010; **6**(1): 85–95.

Bazil CW. Nocturnal seizures and the effects of anticonvulsants on sleep. *Curr Neurol Neurosci Rep* 2008; **8**(2): 149–54.

Boeve BF. Update on the diagnosis and management of sleep disturbances in dementia. *Sleep Med Clin* 2008; **3**(3): 347–60.

Caminero A, Bartolome M. Sleep disturbances in multiple sclerosis. *J Neurol Sci* 2011; **309**(1–2): 86–91.

Chokroverty S. Sleep and breathing in neuromuscular disorders. *Handb Clin Neurol* 2011; **99**: 1087–108.

Dauvilliers Y. Insomnia in patients with neurodegenerative conditions. *Sleep Med* 2007; **8**(Suppl 4): S27–34.

Derry C. Nocturnal frontal lobe epilepsy vs parasomnias. *Curr Treat Options Neurol* 2012; **14**(5): 451–63.

Diederich NJ, McIntyre DJ. Sleep disorders in Parkinson's disease: many causes, few therapeutic options. *J Neurol Sci* 2012; **314**(1–2): 12–19.

Eriksson SH. Epilepsy and sleep. *Curr Opin Neurol* 2011; **24**(2): 171–6.

Hermann DM, Bassetti CL. Sleep-related breathing and sleep-wake disturbances in ischemic stroke. *Neurology* 2009; **73**(16): 1313–22.

Korner Y, Meindorfner C, Möller J, et al. Predictors of sudden onset of sleep in Parkinson's disease. *Mov Disord* 2004; **19**(11): 1298–305.

Li Y, Munger K, Batool-Anwar S, et al. Association of multiple sclerosis with restless legs syndrome and other sleep disorders in women. *Neurology* 2012; **78**(19): 1500–6.

Manni R, Terzaghi M. Comorbidity between epilepsy and sleep disorders. *Epilepsy Res* 2010; **90**(3): 171–7.

Salami O, Lyketsos C, Rao V. Treatment of sleep disturbance in Alzheimer's dementia. *Int J Geriatr Psychiatry* 2011; **26**(8): 771–82.

Wallace DM, Ramos AR, Rundek T. Sleep disorders and stroke. *Int J Stroke* 2012; **7**(3): 231–42.

Zesiewicz TA, Sullivan K, Arnulf I, et al. Practice Parameter: treatment of nonmotor symptoms of Parkinson disease: report of the Quality Standards Subcommittee of the American Academy of Neurology. *Neurology* 2010; **74**(11): 924–31.

14

Cognition, Driving, and Sleep

Makoto Kawai, MD

Department of Neurology, Methodist Neurological Institute,
Weill Cornell Medical College, USA

Introduction

We know that the brain requires sleep because all of us have experienced sleep deprivation whether due to travel, childcare, or school/work projects. However, the severity of impact on our vulnerable cognitive function has been underrecognized. Little attention was paid to this area until significant accidents likely related to sleep deprivation began to be reported. Humans generally tend to underestimate the impact of sleep deprivation on their function. This poor recognition, in addition to the cognitive decline itself, contributes to the many accidents that have been reported, including motor vehicle crashes and occupational accidents.[1] The correlation of cognition and sleep has been studied among subjects with sleep deprivation.

In recent times, growing attention has been paid to the cognitive performance of patients with obstructive sleep apnea (OSA). In addition to the excessive daytime sleepiness, several other cognitive dysfunctions have been reported in association with the sleep-disordered breathing.[2] This chapter will also attempt to review the brain localization of these sleep-related symptoms.

Acute sleep deprivation

Cognitive dysfunction related to sleep deprivation has been studied and a wide variety of cognitive dysfunctions have been reported. Most cognitive functions worsen with sleep deprivation, especially due to the exaggerated fatigue phenomenon.[3] This phenomenon is observed more prominently when the test battery becomes longer and more complicated. However, regardless of the fatigue phenomenon,

some cognitive functions appear more sensitive than others to sleep loss. For instance, the functions of the prefrontal cortex have been reported to be more vulnerable in sleep deprivation.[4]

Functional neuroimaging techniques, including functional magnetic resonance imaging (fMRI) and positron emission tomography (PET), are helping to delineate the localization of the cognitive dysfunction in the brain related to sleep deprivation.[5] For instance, PET studies showed combination of areas of decreased and increased glucose metabolism after acute sleep deprivation. Decreased glucose metabolism was found in the thalamus, basal ganglia, cerebellum, and prefrontal, temporal, and parietal lobes. Increased glucose metabolism was found in the visual cortex.[5]

Cortical dysfunctions due to sleep deprivation can be classified into several groups. The most common symptom to occur after sleep deprivation is sleepiness. This represents the instability of the awake state. The next most common cognitive difficulties are issues with attention and executive function, followed by cognitive dysfunctions other than executive functions. Memory, emotion, and reward are included in this last group. We will cover each of these areas in turn.

Sleepiness

Sleepiness is a subjective and very common symptom of sleep deprivation. Sleepiness can be evaluated with several sleepiness scales, including the Epworth Sleepiness Scale (ESS) or Stanford Sleepiness Scale (SSS).[6,7] The Epworth Scale measures sleepiness in "the recent past" whereas the Standford Scale measures current sleepiness.

Sleep Medicine in Neurology, First Edition. Edited by Douglas B. Kirsch.
© 2014 John Wiley & Sons, Ltd. Published 2014 by John Wiley & Sons, Ltd.

Sleepiness also can be measured objectively via the Multiple Sleep Latency Test (MSLT) or Maintenance of Wakefulness Test (MWT).[8,9] In these laboratory-based studies that are typically performed in the daytime, sleep latency is measured as a parameter of sleepiness. For the MSLT, a sleep latency of less than 8 min is considered part of the diagnostic criteria for narcolepsy. For the MWT, a sleep latency less than 8 min is also considered abnormal; a test result above 8 min but below 40 min (in a 40-min MWT) is of unclear clinical significance. Sleep latency represents how quickly the patient falls asleep without effort to stay awake during the MSLT and with effort to stay awake during the MWT. There is some correlation between the subjective sleepiness scales and sleep latency in objective physiological studies, though the strength of that correlation is less strong than one might expect.

As subjective sleepiness scales are influenced by interindividual variation in recognition of sleepiness or cultural background differences (i.e. items regarding sleepiness while driving in the ESS may not be relevant for those who do not drive), utilizing these scales to compare sleepiness across different populations requires extra caution. In contrast, the MSLT or MWT is a more objective parameter, not influenced by individual differences in recognition or cultural background.

When using a cognitive performance test, sleepiness can be observed via very brief periods of sleep, also known as microsleeps. These symptoms are observed as a lapse of responsiveness or increased errors of commission, especially when the person has to make great effort to stay awake.[10] The phenomenon of increased errors of commission is hypothesized as a symptom of compensation. In other words, this represents a balance between the homeostatic drive to fall asleep and resistance from an awake-promoting mechanism.[3]

Though the MSLT and MWT are currently recognized as the gold standard for measuring sleepiness, these studies show only the objective result of sleepiness. It is reasonable to try to observe sleepiness more directly with neuroimaging studies. fMRI study has shown reduced activity in the prefrontal cortex after sleep deprivation in a serial subtraction task.[11] But in a verbal learning task, the prefrontal cortex and parietal cortex were more activated after sleep deprivation.[12] Interestingly, activation of the prefrontal cortex was positively correlated with subjective sleepiness, whereas activation in a parietal cortex was correlated with preservation of near-normal verbal learning. These patterns of increase and decrease in cerebral activation most likely represent compensatory adaptations, in which other parts of brain not normally activated are recruited to compensate for the reduced function of the brain are typically activated in a certain task. In this case, compensatory adaptation results in more activation in the prefrontal cortex with sleep deprivation, indicating a compensation process in response to the increased homeostatic drive for sleep. On the other hand, activation in a parietal lobe with sleep deprivation suggests an adaptation process to support the decreased function of other areas of the cortex.

These patterns of compensatory adaptation have task-specific differences.[11,13] Level of difficulty modulates the cerebral response as well.[14] Sleepiness is most likely a subjective symptom of these complicated processes of compensatory adaptation.

Attention and executive functions

The next most common cognitive function affected by sleep deprivation is attention. The Psychomotor Vigilance Test (PVT) is often utilized for evaluation of attention, as there are few learning effects due to the simplicity of the test. Clear correlation has been demonstrated between the number of lapses during the test and the duration of sleep deprivation (Figure 14.1).[15]

It may be difficult to distinguish microsleeps and dysfunction in attention because both can possibly cause a lapse in response, unless a neurophysiological study is performed simultaneously with the PVT.

Interindividual differences also contribute to the difficulty of making a neuroimaging study a generalized parameter of sleepiness. In fMRI studies activation of the frontoparietal region was more prominent in the group that was less vulnerable to the effects of sleep deprivation than the group that was more vulnerable.[16] This finding suggests that more activated compensatory adaptation contributes less vulnerability to sleep deprivation.

Other executive functions, including verbal learning, working memory, non-verbal and verbal recognition tasks, also deteriorate with sleep deprivation. In a working memory task with sleep deprivation, a fMRI study revealed decreased activation in the parietal region but increased activation in prefrontal and thalamic regions in

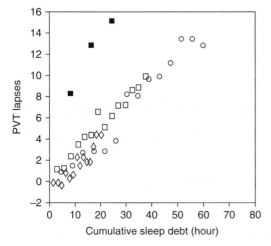

Figure 14.1 Lapses of PVT increase proportionally to the amount of sleep debt and do not reach plateau for subjects in the 8 hours (◊), 6 hours (□), and 4 hours (○) chronic sleep period conditions across 14 days and in the 0 hour (■) sleep condition across 3 days. Van Dongen HP, Maislin G, Mullington JM, Dinges DF. The cumulative cost of additional wakefulness: dose-response effects on neurobehavioural functions and sleep physiology from chronic restriction and total sleep deprivation. Sleep 2003; 26: 117–26.

more complex tasks.[17] This is another example of compensatory adaptation.

Cortical function other than executive functions

Memory

Acute sleep deprivation impairs visual short-term memory. fMRI study reveals a reduction in parietal and extrastriatal activation.[18] There is also a report of a significant decrease in hippocampal activity during episodic memory testing with sleep deprivation.[19] Functional connectivity analysis establishes that sleep deprivation alters connectivity between the hippocampus and basic alertness networks of the brainstem and thalamus during a memory consolidation task.[19]

Sleep deprivation can also alter the slow-learning processes of memory consolidation. Maquet et al. performed a study utilizing a visuomotor task and fMRI. They trained participants to perform visuomotor tasks and then evaluated the effect of sleep after learning. The group who had been sleep deprived had reduction of activation in the area of the superior temporal sulcus which correlated with their decline in task performance.[20]

Emotion and reward

Functional MRI study revealed that recollection of negative stimuli with sleep deprivation elicited higher responses in the amygdala and occipital area. In contrast, no difference in brain responses was observed with recollection of positive stimuli.[21]

Sleep deprivation elevated expectations of higher reward on a gambling task, as nucleus accumbens activation increased with risky choices, and in the insular and orbitofrontal cortices, neural responses to losses are attenuated.[22] Thus, the typical trip to Las Vegas may not be optimal, as gamblers with sleep deprivation appear to have an altered expectation of reward and smaller response to losses, along with deteriorated executive functions.

Chronic sleep deprivation

After sleep restriction to 40% of typical sleep amounts for five nights, progressive deterioration in performance on a vigilance and simple reaction time performance task is observed.[23] The number of lapses in the PVT continues to increase even at the 14th day of sleep restriction. However, sleepiness as measured by the SSS plateaus around 4–6 days (Figure 14.2).[15] This combination of findings suggests that subjective sleepiness is not always in a linear correlation with dysfunction of attention; in other words, humans continue to perform worse with chronic sleep deprivation even though we believe that our sleepiness is not worsening. Another study showed that sleep restriction to 4 hours for 1 week caused decline in performance of the PVT to levels similar to those seen with total sleep deprivation for 24 hours.[15] Also, the speed of response in the PVT continues to decrease over a week of sleep deprivation.[23] Even though the impact of chronic sleep deprivation is significant and cumulative, the time required for recovery is relatively short, i.e. 1–2 days for attention measured with the PVT.[23]

Accidents and safety

Annual economic impact related to accidents seconday to sleep deprivation has been reported to be as high as $43–56 billion.[24]

Work-hour regulation in the medical field

One of the biggest changes in modern medical training is the introduction of work-hour regulation during training of physicians. Libby Zion's case in New York drew attention to the increased risk of medical errors in the sleep-deprived physician in

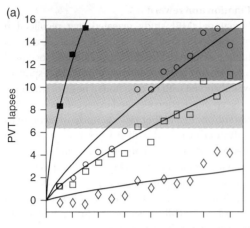
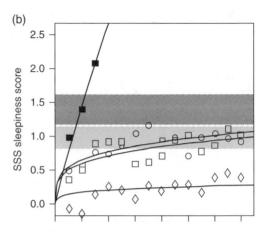

Figure 14.2 Each line in graph A shows a different rate of increase in lapses of PVT and graph B shows subjective sleepiness on the SSS for subjects in the 8 hours (◊), 6 hours (□), and 4 hours (○) chronic sleep period conditions across 14 days and in the 0 hour (■) sleep condition across 3 days. The rate increases with the severity of sleep deprivation and lapses continue to increase proportional to duration of sleep deprivation in all groups. The SSS reaches a plateau in chronic sleep deprivation groups but not in a total sleep deprivation group. Van Dongen HP, Maislin G, Mullington JM, Dinges DF. The cumulative cost of additional wakefulness: dose-response effects on neurobehavioural functions and sleep physiology from chronic restriction and total sleep deprivation. Sleep 2003; 26: 117–26.

training.[25,26] One study demonstrated that postcall residents with acute sleep deprivation perform at the same level as those with a blood alcohol concentration of 0.04–0.05% in neurobehavioral tests.[27] These findings contributed to the justification for duty-hour regulation in medical training by the Accreditation Council of Graduate Medical Education.[28] Despite criticism of these regulations, the high arousal and attention level required for the complexity of medical issues and a zero tolerance rate for errors appear to justify the regulation. In addition, beyond work performance, there is also the risk of motor vehicle accidents when sleepy physicians are driving home after a call night.

There are several factors that need to be taken into consideration when deriving these regulations. One is the variety of vulnerability to sleep deprivation in the target populations. The other is the dissociation of sleepiness and performance with sleep deprivation. In other words, subjective sleepiness may not be a good parameter for monitoring performance. Thus, the regulation should be created to be effective for the most vulnerable members of the resident population and should not be modified based on reported subjective sleepiness, and one must aware that current regulation for resident work hours may not be stringent enough for individual residents.

★ TIPS AND TRICKS

For residents taking overnight calls:

- try not to start on call with sleep debt
- try to take a short sleep/nap if possible, especially between 2.00 am and 5.00 am
- try not to make any complicated decisions on a postcall day, even if you do not feel sleepy
- try not to drive between 2.00 pm and 5.00 pm on a postcall day, especially for long distances
- take a short nap between 2.00 pm and 5.00 pm for less than 30 min on a postcall day
- sleep in the evening on a postcall day.

Cognition and obstructive sleep apnea

This area has been investigated extensively. OSA has a high prevalence of 2–4% in adults and 1–3% in children.[29,30] The multiple reports of car, train, and plane accidents potentially related to excessive daytime sleepiness from OSA have drawn the attention of the media and government agencies. In addition to excessive daytime sleepiness, there are many other cognitive functions that function less well in patients with OSA.[2]

For the majority of patients with OSA, it appears likely that the cognitive deficits are related to sleep fragmentation, increased breathing effort, and intermittent blood gas abnormalities (hypoxia, hypercarbia).[2] Similar to the sleep deprivation studies, executive dysfunction from a deficit in the prefrontal cortex has been reported in patients with OSA.[2] Also cognitive difficulties other than executive function have been reported.[2] In addition to the direct effect of OSA, one indirect effect is an increase in stroke risk. Strokes may in turn contribute to cognitive decline.[31]

In contrast to sleep deprivation, the biggest concern about cognitive decline in OSA is the possibility that the deficits are irreversible. Several neuroimaging studies of patients with OSA display morphological changes of gray matter loss in a widespread area in addition to the functional decline.[32, 33] There is also a report of diffuse bilateral gray matter loss observed in parietal and frontal cortices as well as in bilateral parahippocampal gyri.[33] These morphological findings did not reverse after optimal continuous positive airway pressure (CPAP) treatment.[34] Proton MR spectroscopy study demonstrates neuronal loss in frontal white matter in patients with OSA.[35] A fMRI study reveals a persistent lack of dorsolateral prefrontal activation in CPAP-treated patients with OSA when performing a working memory task, even after complete clinical recovery.[36] Thus it appears that recurrent hypoxia and sleep fragmentation may play a role in developing persistent brain abnormalities in both function and morphology.

Driving and sleep

In several studies, patients with OSA demonstrate an increased odds ratio for having a motor vehicle accident, being 1.2–4.9 times more likely to have accidents than the control general population.[37] Multiple factors correlated with risk of motor vehicle accidents included Body Mass Index (BMI), Apnea-Hypopnea Index (AHI), oxygen saturation, and possibly daytime sleepiness based on the ESS.[37]

Sleep deprivation is another cause of potential driving accidents. Using simulated driving markers such as lane variability, accuracy or reaction time after more than 16 hours of sleep deprivation has been reported to be similar to that of subjects with a blood alcohol content of 0.05–0.1%.[38,39] When comparing the three factors of sleep deprivation, OSA, and alcohol, patients subjected to sleep deprivation

who also had OSA showed progressive deterioration of performance through the driving task, whereas patients who had taken alcohol had an impaired steering error which was relatively stable during the task.[40]

There are several studies which have attempted to detect drowsy driving, with the eventual goal of being able to prevent it. Several studies have shown bursts of alpha activity diffusely or in central regions on electroencephalogram (EEG) before subjects make driving errors.[41,42] The alpha activity is clearly different from the occipital dominant rhythm in its distribution. This finding has been correlated with drowsiness and errors when the subject is applying maximum effort to stay awake. Thus this activity may not be considered as an awake phenomenon.

Circadian rhythms affect driving performance and the incidence of motor vehicle accidents. Connor et al. reported a five-fold higher incidence of motor vehicle accidents between 2.00 am and 5.00 am compared with other times of day.[43] In those early morning hours, melatonin secretion reaches its peak and core body temperature is at its minimum level.

In a report on driving performance, especially speed control, Lenne et al. revealed deterioration in that performance around 2.00 pm to 5.00 pm, corresponding to the mid-afternoon circadian temperature dip, in addition to early morning deterioration between 2.00 am and 5.00 am.[44] The performance deficits were more prominent in low stimulus driving (i.e. highway and rural driving).[45]

Neuroimaging has been performed in driving simulator studies, during which pedal variables correlated with increased activation in the motor areas of the brain, and steering was associated with the cerebellum.[46] However, effects of sleep deprivation or OSA in driving with neuroimaging still need to be investigated.

In the sleep clinic, questions often arise about driving safely, particularly in patients with known sleep disorders. In my opinion, physicians should include several factors, in addition to the legal restrictions provided by the licensing authority. The most important thing to emphasize is that limiting sleep can lead to increased risk of motor vehicle accidents, particularly if there is an underlying sleep disorder. Also, taking alcohol increases the risk for accidents, especially when combined with sleep deprivation or a disorder of sleep fragmentation.[38–40,47,48]

> ⚠ **CAUTION**
>
> - Don't drink and drive. This is especially true when one is sleep deprived or has untreated sleep disorders, such as OSA.
> - Avoid sleep deprivation when OSA is present.
> - Be aware of the length of the journey. The longer the drive, the worse the driving will be if you are sleep deprived and OSA.
> - Treatment of OSA is important both to minimize motor vehicle accidents and to limit cognitive impact.
> - Do not trust your subjective assessment of sleepiness, as your actual performance tends to be worse than you suspect.

Conclusion

Cognition and sleep are closely related. We can demonstrate this by disturbing normal sleep via different methods. Examples include acute sleep deprivation, chronic sleep deprivation, and untreated OSA. Attention, executive functions, and other cognitive processes are affected by these abnormal sleep conditions. One difference between sleep deprivation and obstructive sleep apnea is its reversibility. While almost all of the cognitive deficit caused by sleep deprivation is reversible by obtaining the correct amount of sleep, there is evidence that at least some of the deficits that occur in patients with OSA are irreversible.

Sleepiness can cause motor vehicle and job-related accidents. Especially in the medical field, sleep deprivation has been proven to cause a decline in cognitive function. Both sleep deprivation and OSA cause progressive deterioration related to driving distance, whereas alcohol showed a consistency of poor performance throughout driving tasks. Driving performance is also influenced by circadian rhythms. During drowsy driving, unique alpha burst activity has been reported before making errors.

References

1. Horne J, Reyner L. Vehicle accidents related to sleep: a review. *Occup Environ Med* 1999; **56**: 289–94.
2. Beebe DW, Gozal D. Obstructive sleep apnea and the prefrontal cortex: towards a comprehensive model linking nocturnal upper airway obstruction to daytime cognitive and behavioral deficits. *J Sleep Res* 2002; **11**: 1–16.
3. Goel N, Rao H, Durmer JS, Dinges DF. Neurocognitive consequences of sleep deprivation. *Semin Neurol* 2009; **29**: 320–39.
4. Horne JA. Human sleep, sleep loss and behaviour. Implications for the prefrontal cortex and psychiatric disorder. *Br J Psychiatry* 1993; **162**: 413–19.
5. Dang-Vu TT, Desseilles M, Petit D, Mazza S, Montplaisir J, Maquet P. Neuroimaging in sleep medicine. *Sleep Med* 2007; **8**: 349–72.
6. Johns MW. A new method for measuring daytime sleepiness: the Epworth sleepiness scale. *Sleep* 1991; **14**: 540–5.
7. Hoddes E, Zarcone V, Smythe H, Phillips R, Dement WC. Quantification of sleepiness: a new approach. *Psychophysiology* 1973; **10**: 431–6.
8. Richardson GS, Carskadon MA, Flagg W, van den Hoed J, Dement WC, Mitler MM. Excessive daytime sleepiness in man: multiple sleep latency measurement in narcoleptic and control subjects. *Electroencephalogr Clin Neurophysiol* 1978; **45**: 621–7.
9. Mitler MM, Gujavarty KS, Browman CP. Maintenance of wakefulness test: a polysomnographic technique for evaluation treatment efficacy in patients with excessive somnolence. *Electroencephalogr Clin Neurophysiol* 1982; **53**: 658–61.
10. Lim J, Dinges DF. Sleep deprivation and vigilant attention. *Ann N Y Acad Sci* 2008; **1129**: 305–22.
11. Drummond SP, Brown GG, Stricker JL, Buxton RB, Wong EC, Gillin JC. Sleep deprivation-induced reduction in cortical functional response to serial subtraction. *Neuroreport* 1999; **10**: 3745–8.
12. Drummond SP, Brown GG, Gillin JC, Stricker JL, Wong EC, Buxton RB. Altered brain response to verbal learning following sleep deprivation. *Nature* 2000; **403**: 655–7.
13. Mu Q, Nahas Z, Johnson KA, et al. Decreased cortical response to verbal working memory following sleep deprivation. *Sleep* 2005; **28**: 55–67.
14. Drummond SP, Brown GG, Salamat JS, Gillin JC. Increasing task difficulty facilitates the cerebral compensatory response to total sleep deprivation. *Sleep* 2004; **27**: 445–51.

15. Van Dongen HP, Maislin G, Mullington JM, Dinges DF. The cumulative cost of additional wakefulness: dose–response effects on neurobehavioral functions and sleep physiology from chronic sleep restriction and total sleep deprivation. *Sleep* 2003; **26**: 117–26.

16. Mu Q, Mishory A, Johnson KA, et al. Decreased brain activation during a working memory task at rested baseline is associated with vulnerability to sleep deprivation. *Sleep* 2005; **28**: 433–46.

17. Chee MW, Choo WC. Functional imaging of working memory after 24 hr of total sleep deprivation. *J Neurosci* 2004; **24**: 4560–7.

18. Chee MW, Chuah YM. Functional neuroimaging and behavioral correlates of capacity decline in visual short-term memory after sleep deprivation. *Proc Natl Acad Sci USA* 2007; **104**: 9487–92.

19. Yoo SS, Hu PT, Gujar N, Jolesz FA, Walker MP. A deficit in the ability to form new human memories without sleep. *Nat Neurosci* 2007; **10**: 385–92.

20. Maquet P, Schwartz S, Passingham R, Frith C. Sleep-related consolidation of a visuomotor skill: brain mechanisms as assessed by functional magnetic resonance imaging. *J Neurosci* 2003; **23**: 1432–40.

21. Sterpenich V, Albouy G, Boly M, et al. Sleep-related hippocampo-cortical interplay during emotional memory recollection. *PLoS Biol* 2007; **5**: e282.

22. Venkatraman V, Chuah YM, Huettel SA, Chee MW. Sleep deprivation elevates expectation of gains and attenuates response to losses following risky decisions. *Sleep* 2007; **30**: 603–9.

23. Belenky G, Wesensten NJ, Thorne DR, et al. Patterns of performance degradation and restoration during sleep restriction and subsequent recovery: a sleep dose–response study. *J Sleep Res* 2003; **12**: 1–12.

24. Leger D. The cost of sleep-related accidents: a report for the National Commission on Sleep Disorders Research. *Sleep* 1994; **17**: 84–93.

25. The Libby Zion case. *Ann Intern Med* 1991; **115**: 985–6.

26. Asch DA, Parker RM. The Libby Zion case. One step forward or two steps backward? *N Engl J Med* 1988; **318**: 771–5.

27. Arnedt JT, Owens J, Crouch M, Stahl J, Carskadon MA. Neurobehavioral performance of residents after heavy night call vs after alcohol ingestion. *JAMA* 2005; **294**: 1025–33.

28. Philibert I, Friedmann P, Williams WT. New requirements for resident duty hours. *JAMA* 2002; **288**: 1112–14.

29. Young T, Palta M, Dempsey J, Skatrud J, Weber S, Badr S. The occurrence of sleep-disordered breathing among middle-aged adults. *N Engl J Med* 1993; **328**: 1230–5.

30. Lumeng JC, Chervin RD. Epidemiology of pediatric obstructive sleep apnea. *Proc Am Thorac Soc* 2008; **5**: 242–52.

31. Dyken ME, Somers VK, Yamada T, Ren ZY, Zimmerman MB. Investigating the relationship between stroke and obstructive sleep apnea. *Stroke* 1996; **27**: 401–7.

32. Yaouhi K, Bertran F, Clochon P, et al. A combined neuropsychological and brain imaging study of obstructive sleep apnea. *J Sleep Res* 2009; **18**: 36–48.

33. Macey PM, Henderson LA, Macey KE, et al. Brain morphology associated with obstructive sleep apnea. *Am J Respir Crit Care Med* 2002; **166**: 1382–7.

34. O'Donoghue FJ, Briellmann RS, Rochford PD, et al. Cerebral structural changes in severe obstructive sleep apnea. *Am J Respir Crit Care Med* 2005; **171**: 1185–90.

35. Alchanatis M, Deligiorgis N, Zias N, et al. Frontal brain lobe impairment in obstructive sleep apnoea: a proton MR spectroscopy study. *Eur Respir J* 2004; **24**: 980–6.

36. Thomas RJ, Rosen BR, Stern CE, Weiss JW, Kwong KK. Functional imaging of working memory in obstructive sleep-disordered breathing. *J Appl Physiol* 2005; **98**: 2226–34.

37. Tregear S, Reston J, Schoelles K, Phillips B. Obstructive sleep apnea and risk of motor vehicle crash: systematic review and meta-analysis. *J Clin Sleep Med* 2009; **5**: 573–81.

38. Williamson AM, Feyer AM. Moderate sleep deprivation produces impairments in cognitive and motor performance equivalent to legally prescribed levels of alcohol intoxication. *Occup Environ Med* 2000; **57**: 649–55.

39. Dawson D, Reid K. Fatigue, alcohol and performance impairment. *Nature* 1997; **388**: 235.

40. Hack MA, Choi SJ, Vijayapalan P, Davies RJ, Stradling JR. Comparison of the effects of sleep deprivation, alcohol and obstructive sleep apnoea (OSA) on simulated steering performance. *Respir Med* 2001; **95**: 594–601.

41. Torsvall L, Akerstedt T. Sleepiness on the job: continuously measured EEG changes in train drivers. *Electroencephalogr Clin Neurophysiol* 1987; **66**: 502–11.

42. Papadelis C, Chen Z, Kourtidou-Papadeli C, et al. Monitoring sleepiness with on-board electrophysiological recordings for preventing sleep-deprived traffic accidents. *Clin Neurophysiol* 2007; **118**: 1906–22.

43. Connor J, Norton R, Ameratunga S, et al. Driver sleepiness and risk of serious injury to car occupants: population based case control study. *BMJ* 2002; **324**: 1125.

44. Lenne MG, Triggs TJ, Redman JR. Time of day variations in driving performance. *Accid Anal Prev* 1997; **29**: 431–7.

45. Reimer B, d'Ambrosio LA, Coughlin JF. Secondary analysis of time of day on simulated driving performance. *J Safety Res* 2007; **38**: 563–70.

46. Carvalho KN, Pearlson GD, Astur RS, Calhoun VD. Simulated driving and brain imaging: combining behavior, brain activity, and virtual reality. *CNS Spectr* 2006; **11**: 52–62.

47. Vakulin A, Baulk SD, Catcheside PG, et al. Effects of moderate sleep deprivation and low-dose alcohol on driving simulator performance and perception in young men. *Sleep* 2007; **30**: 1327–33.

48. Fairclough SH, Graham R. Impairment of driving performance caused by sleep deprivation or alcohol: a comparative study. *Hum Factors* 1999; **41**: 118–28.

15

Pediatric Sleep Medicine

Shalini Paruthi, MD

Saint Louis University School of Medicine and Pediatric Sleep and Research Center, SSM Cardinal Glennon Children's Medical Center, USA

Introduction

Many children suffering from neurological conditions have sleep complaints such as insomnia, awakenings, or excessive sleepiness. Sleep disorders are commonly seen in patients with headaches, epilepsy, traumatic brain injury or concussions, developmental delay, neuromuscular disorders, hypersomnia or narcolepsy, parasomnias, neuropathy, and hyperactivity or behavior disturbances. Thus it is important in comprehensive neurological care to also obtain a sleep history, as treating the underlying sleep condition may improve the neurological disorder. Children may develop sleep disorders seen in patients of any age, or a unique pediatric sleep disorder, such as behavioral insomnia of childhood, limit setting or sleep onset association disorder.

This chapter will discuss a detailed sleep medicine evaluation, with elaboration of sleep onset insomnia, sleep maintenance insomnia, hypersomnia, and nocturnal motor events. Additional sleep topics will be briefly covered with emphasis on the key differences in evaluation, diagnosis, and treatment between adults and children. More in-depth details of diagnosis, evaluation, and treatment can be found in the accompanying chapters on each topic.

The major classifications of sleep disorders include insomnia, breathing disorders, hypersomnias, circadian rhythm disturbances, parasomnias, and sleep-related movements.

Often the sleep problem has been long standing, with resultant exhausted sleep-deprived parents who have already tried "family" and "internet" remedies. Thus a family-friendly setting can help a child (and parent) feel at ease in clinic to facilitate the exchange of information.

Furthermore, it is a common belief that simply correcting sleep hygiene will resolve the majority of sleep complaints in children. Sleep hygiene is unlikely to be the sole cause of insomnia, but it is still important to review and emphasize. If behavior change recommendations do not fully resolve the sleep complaints, then a more in-depth evaluation for a medical or sleep disorder is indicated.

A key portion of any sleep discussion involves defining sleep expectations (helping parents understand what is normal).

1. "Sleeping through the night" for an infant is 5–6 hours per commonly held definition; this is usually achieved once a child is at least 12–14 pounds in weight, and often about 6 months in age. It may occur sooner.

2. Most children cannot sleep more than 10 hours consistently at night without food or drink. See Table 15.1 for optimal suggested hours of sleep by age.

3. Parents often need help setting the bedtime in toddlers or grade school children. Parents should first choose the wake-up time, then count backwards the age-appropriate hours of sleep for the child. For example, if a 7-year-old child has to wake up at 6.30 am to get ready for the school bus that comes at 7.15 am, then counting 10 hours previous determines the 8.30 pm bedtime. On the other hand, for a 4-year-old child who needs to awaken at 8 am because his mother leaves him at daycare at 9 am, where he

Sleep Medicine in Neurology, First Edition. Edited by Douglas B. Kirsch.
© 2014 John Wiley & Sons, Ltd. Published 2014 by John Wiley & Sons, Ltd.

Table 15.1 Optimal suggested hours of sleep by age

Age	Hours of sleep
Infants (up to age 1 year)	10–16 hours of sleep in small 2–4-hours increments
Toddlers (age 1–5 years)	11–14 hours of sleep, including the daytime nap
Grade school (kindergarten to 8th grade)	9–10 hours overnight
High school (9th to 12th grade)	9.25–8.5 hours overnight

takes a 2-hours nap, then a bedtime at 10 pm may be appropriate. Giving this child an earlier bedtime might actually cause insomnia if he is given too much opportunity to be in bed.

Sleep onset insomnia

The most commonly encountered medical causes of pediatric sleep onset insomnia are restless legs syndrome (or variant), anxiety, circadian rhythm disturbance in the form of delayed sleep phase disorder, and behavioral resistance. Furthermore, medical disorders strongly associated with insomnia include autism, Asperger's syndrome, autistic spectrum disorder, pervasive developmental disorder, oppositional defiant disorder, developmental delay, and cerebral palsy. Behavioral insomnia is also discussed in this section.

Restless legs syndrome (RLS) and RLS variants

In this disorder, the essential diagnostic criteria are the same as for adults with the additional criteria that the child can describe the urge to move or the uncomfortable sensation in their own words. The four essential criteria include an urge to move or uncomfortable sensation in the legs, worse in the evenings or night, worse with inactivity or rest, and improvement with movement. The diagnosis can also be made if the child meets all four major criteria *and* has two of the three following criteria: a sleep disturbance, a first-degree family member with RLS, or elevated periodic limb movement (PLM) index seen on in-laboratory polysomnography.

Suspect RLS-variant in a child who meets at least two of the four major criteria. Of note, RLS and its variants are a clinical diagnosis. An in-laboratory polysomnogram is not typically required to make the diagnosis, unless looking for the elevated periodic limb movement index.

In practice, a parent often describes the child as restless, kicks when falling asleep, and tosses and turns through the night. While 2% of children meet all the essential criteria for RLS, an estimated 17% of children are restless sleepers, and frequently improve when evaluated and treated as RLS. Evidence is increasing between the overlap of "growing pains" and RLS. In children, eliciting the symptoms of RLS may be difficult due to their verbal skills, their ability to perceive and describe the sensation and their inability to know or realize they are not supposed to have uncomfortable sensations. Although open-ended questions are recommended in healthcare, it may be prudent to ask "multiple choice" questions of young children. For example, if a child answers 'yes' to questions on leg pains, then the next question might be "Does it hurt more in the morning or afternoon at school, in the evening or at night?" Interestingly, though the standard RLS criteria include leg pains which are worse at evening or nighttime, occasionally parents of children with RLS report their child also has morning leg pains upon awakening that resolve quickly.

The pathophysiology of pediatric RLS is presumed to be similar to that of adults with a defect in the production or transport of dopamine, for which iron is a required co-factor for the rate-limiting enzyme tyrosine hydroxylase.

First-line therapy begins with iron supplementation, unless contraindicated due to hemochromatosis or other iron metabolism disorder. It is recommended to check a ferritin level. If ferritin is <50 ng/mL then liquid elemental iron supplementation is recommended at a dose of 1–2 mg/kg dosed twice a day, with vitamin C, such as juice, for children unable to swallow tablets. Additionally, ferrous sulfate 325 mg (65 mg elemental) tablets can be considered daily or twice daily, to reach a target of 1–2 mg/kg bid. (See Table 15.2 for additional forms of commonly available iron preparations.) The most common side-effects to be discussed with patients include flatus, constipation, and stool color changes (black or dark green). A prescription for polyethylene glycol (Miralax) is often given concurrently. Ferritin levels may be checked at 12-week intervals (no sooner than 6-week intervals) and the iron dose adjusted up or down accordingly.

Table 15.2 Forms of commonly used iron preparations

Liquid	Chew tablets	Swallow tablets
Ferrous sulfate drops 15 mg/1 mL = elemental iron 15 mg/1 mL	Flintstones (or generic) complete hard chewable tablets contain 18 mg of iron per chew tablet	Ferrous sulfate 325 mg = elemental iron 65 mg
Ferrous sulfate elixir 220 mg/5 mL = elemental iron 44 mg/5 mL		Ferrous gluconate 225 mg = elemental iron 27 mg
Polyvisol with iron by Enfamil elemental iron 10 mg/1 mL solution	Nearly all gummy vitamins do not contain iron	Over-the-counter (on the shelf) iron is found in various dosage amounts (usually listed by elemental iron in milligrams)

☆ **TIPS AND TRICKS**

How to get children to take ferrous sulfate liquid

1. Measure out the appropriate amount of liquid iron into a small medicine cup, add one sip of the child's favorite juice, and get them to drink through a short straw. Children find this funny and it avoids the bitter taste of iron as well as avoiding staining of teeth. If tooth discoloration occurs, baking soda (in toothpaste or on toothbrush) removes the stain.
2. Measure out the appropriate amount of liquid iron into a tablespoon, then add apple sauce or other flavored sauce.

☆ **TIPS AND TRICKS**

Avoid gastrointestinal side-effects of iron
Prescribe Miralax prn at the same time prescription is provided for ferrous sulfate. Initial Miralax dosing is to start with one-quarter capful daily until the child has a soft, formed bowel movement, without abdominal pain. This can be increased or decreased as needed to keep bowel movements soft and formed.

✋ **CAUTION**

Iron safety
Safety of iron storage out of the reach of children should be discussed with parents; iron is the most common cause of poisoning

death in children under age 6 years. Symptoms of severe nausea, vomiting, and diarrhea may begin within hours if a child ingests as little as >10 mg/kg at once; lethal doses of iron vary per child based on weight.

As there are currently no Federal Drug Administration (FDA)-approved medications for RLS in children, second-line off-label therapy is currently with gabapentin or dopamine agonists. Clonazepam has also been used in children, once it has been confirmed the child does not have sleep-disordered breathing.

Gabapentin is generally well tolerated. Safety dosing guidelines are available down to age 2 years. A once-daily dose of 50–100 mg may be taken with dinner or at least 2 hours before the expected onset of symptoms. A rare side-effect specific to children is aggression in addition to the long list of potential side-effects on the package insert.

Alternative second-line off-label therapy includes the dopamine agonists ropinirole, pramipexole, or rotigotine. Review of the child's medication list will help determine if a dopamine agonist may be contraindicated, if the child is already taking other dopamine-mediated medications. The side-effects of nausea, excessive daytime sleepiness, headache, and compulsive behaviors, in addition to those listed in the package insert, should be discussed with parents. In some cases, pramipexole may be crushed and suspended by a compounding pharmacy. Rotigotine is administered through a skin patch. At the time of going to press, rotigotine is under open-label testing in adolescents with RLS between the ages of 13 to 17 years.

> ### Box 15.1 Non-pharmacological treatment options of restless legs syndrome in children
>
> Cook meals in cast iron skillets when possible
> Increase intake of iron-rich foods
> Limit overly vigorous activities before bed (may be difficult with extracurricular activities)
> Wear compression stockings or ace wrap in the evenings (remove before sleep)
> Wear sequential compression devices on the legs for 30 min in the evenings (can be bought commercially)
> Avoid caffeine after 4.00 pm
> Warm bath/shower before bedtime
> Tuck child into bed with socks or blanket that have been warmed in a clothes dryer for 5–10 min

Parents should be advised that they will see noticeable improvements in RLS symptoms 2–8 weeks after initiating iron therapy and may see a response within 1–2 weeks of starting gabapentin or dopamine agonist therapy. By 12 weeks, the parents should note that the child is falling asleep faster, staying asleep longer, and awakening more refreshed, with improvement or resolution of leg pains and parasomnias. Additional benefits of iron and improved sleep reported by parents include increased appetite, growth spurt 4–6 weeks following initiation, increased energy, endurance, and less susceptibility to upper respiratory infections.

See Box 15.1 for non-pharmacological treatment options for children with RLS.

Medical disorders frequently associated with sleep onset insomnia

Children with autistic spectrum disorder (ASD), including autism, Asperger's syndrome, and pervasive developmental disorder, commonly are deficient in melatonin-producing enzymes, and may also secrete melatonin more during the day, rather than at night. Thus, supplemental melatonin near bedtime may be necessary in the treatment of insomnia.

Children with developmental delay or cerebral palsy often have "insomnia" at night due to their "unintentional napping" from limited mobility and static environment throughout the day. This is especially true for children who are wheelchair bound. Sleep may occur at variable times throughout the day, for variable amounts, and thus decrease or eliminate sleep debt at bedtime and overnight.

Melatonin 30–60 min before bedtime, coupled with a consistent bedtime routine, may improve sleep onset at night. Increased physical or occupational therapy, movements and activities during the day may also increase energy expenditure during the day, improving ability to fall asleep at bedtime. An additional recommendation is to carefully screen for a family history of sleep disorders in parents and siblings as the child may have a similar sleep disorder without the ability to communicate symptoms.

Melatonin is not regulated by the FDA and is available over the counter. Due to the lack of regulation, melatonin dosage of each tablet may not be appropriately represented by the packaging label. Most children tolerate a 1–3 mg dose well, 30–45 min before bedtime. Short-acting and controlled-release melatonin formulations are available, and effect typically is greatest on decreasing sleep latency. Melatonin is available as liquid, rapid-dissolving tablets, and swallow tablets. Ramelteon, a melatonin receptor agonist, is available for use in adults but safety and effectiveness have not been established in children.

A polysomnogram is not necessary to make the diagnosis of insomnia, but should be considered if there is suspicion for a co-morbid sleep disorder, such as obstructive sleep apnea.

Circadian rhythm disturbance – delayed sleep phase (DSP) type

During puberty, the circadian rhythm shifts in all children, typically 1 hour later than it had been previously. This change is typically compensated by an hour decrease in sleep need as the child matures and enters high school. However, for a minority of children, the shift can be more extreme, sometimes up to 4 or 8 hours, with sleepiness not occurring until 5.00 or 6.00 am. The most reliable and diagnostic information is often obtained by eliciting bedtimes and wake times during three distinct scenarios: weekdays during the school year, short vacation breaks during the school year, and summer (when there are typically minimal obligations such as school, camps, or work). Diagnostic criteria include delay of the major sleep period in relation to the desired sleep and wake times, the child exhibits normal sleep quality and duration for age when allowed to choose a preferred schedule, and they maintain this delayed, stable phase of entrainment. Maintenance of a sleep log or undergoing actigraphy monitoring (use of a small motion detector worn on wrist or ankle able to distinguish wake and rest) for at least 7 days demonstrates a stable delay of the major sleep period.

Seven to eighteen percent of children have delayed sleep phase disorder. Management includes several interventions: reestablishing the same wake-up time and bedtimes every day including weekends, and 15 min of sun or daylight in the morning to help reset the circadian rhythm. Melatonin may be beneficial, though it often is not necessary. Furthermore, depending on the severity of DSP and the motivation of the child and parent, the child may benefit from chronotherapy, in which the child progressively and dramatically delays their schedule until they end up in a more societally acceptable sleep schedule. A sample schedule for chronotherapy is shown in Table 15.3. Furthermore, cognitive behavioral therapy for insomnia (CBT-I), which includes stimulus control, sleep restriction, cognitive reframing, and relaxation techniques, has also shown efficacy in a research study. CBT-I is

Table 15.3 Chronotherapy schedule – 1 week

Day	Bedtime	Wake-up time
1	4.00 am	12 noon
2	7.00 am	3.00 pm
3	10.00 am	6.00 pm
4	1.00 pm	9.00 pm
5	4.00 pm	12 midnight
6	7.00 pm	3.00 am
7	10.00 pm	7.00 am

Sample schedule for a 15-year-old child who does not regularly feel sleepy or fall asleep until 4.00 am and must get up by 7.00 am for school. Chronotherapy is best done over a short break in the school calendar schedule or the week prior to school start. For chronotherapy to be most effective, parents need to help the child adhere closely to the schedule which will rotate around the clock and induce a slight sleep deprivation. Children should avoid naps to help maximize treatment and maintenance.

typically performed weekly for 4–6 weeks by a sleep physician or sleep psychologist.

Having the child or parent keep a 2-week sleep diary frequently provides the information for a diagnosis of delayed sleep phase. A polysomnogram is not required to make the diagnosis for delayed sleep phase syndrome. However, a sleep study should be considered if there is suspicion for a co-morbid sleep disorder, such as obstructive sleep apnea. Additionally, actigraphy, as described above, can also provide an output displaying the distinct pattern of delayed sleep phase.

Behavioral insomnia of childhood – sleep onset association disorder (BIC-SOAD)

Children require the environment they fall asleep in to be unchanged for the rest of the night. It is normal for children (and adults) to wake up four or more times per night spontaneously. An arousal index of 11 or fewer cortical arousals per hour on sleep electroencephalogram (EEG) is considered normal in children. These several, normal spontaneous awakenings during the night typically involve the child looking around, changing position, and then employing self-soothing skills to fall back to sleep without needing intervention by parents. Sleep association disorder occurs when children require parental or extensive intervention to be able to fall back to sleep after a normal spontaneous awakening. The parent will present to your office stating the child has frequent awakenings at night and takes a long time to put back to sleep for the usual caregiver. Conversely, these children easily fall asleep for other caregivers. BIC-SOAD rarely occurs prior to age 6 months and occurs equally in boys and girls. An example of BIC-SOAD occurs when parents rock a child to sleep, then lays the child down to sleep; a short while later, the child awakens and will only fall back asleep if the intervention of rocking is performed again.

Treatment involves simplifying the environment and bedtime routine so they are easily reproducible if needed during the night hours. Parents must be consistent and persistent nightly. Other specific examples include if a night light or light machine projects images onto the ceiling or wall, these should be left on the entire night. Parents also need to remember to take the light or sound machine that is used nightly whenever they leave the house overnight. Another example: for a child who soothes with a pacifier, placing multiple pacifiers in the crib near the baby's head and hands will ensure a pacifier is within easy reach at all times.

A polysomnogram is not required to make this diagnosis, but a sleep study should be considered for children suspected of co-morbid sleep disorders, such as obstructive sleep apnea.

Behavioral insomnia of childhood – limit setting disorder (BIC-LSD)

Children value routines, so when a parent or caregiver does not set or enforce bedtimes and wake-up times or the bedtime routine, limit setting disorder can occur. Children may stall at bedtime, such as emerging several times from their rooms for "curtain calls." These are frequent requests for a sip of water, another hug or kiss, etc. When parents inconsistently relent to these requests, the situation escalates.

Evaluation of limit setting disorder requires screening for all other medical and sleep disorders that may be causing sleep onset insomnia, including restless legs syndrome. A polysomnogram is not required for the diagnosis, but a sleep study should be ordered if there is suspicion for a co-morbid sleep disorder, such as obstructive sleep apnea.

Once the insomnia is determined to be behavioral in nature, then the parent should be instructed on enforcing good sleep hygiene, setting a bedtime and wake-up time that is similar on all days of the week (less than 1 hour variation), and formally develop a bedtime routine that includes the child's preferences. Then parents must persistently and consistently enforce these new times and routine. In addition, techniques such as extinction, graduated extinction, and bedtime passes may be utilized.

The extinction technique, also known as "crying it out," allows the child to learn to self-soothe without parental intervention, so that with normal spontaneous awakenings at night, the child will not disturb parents. This technique can be difficult for many parents to tolerate. Essentially a parent places their child to sleep in the crib or bed, ensures the child is not ill or at risk for injury, and leaves the room. The child may cry, play, or talk themselves to sleep. Parents only return to check on the child if there is concern for illness or injury.

Graduated extinction is a similar, modified technique and can be used with children aged 2 years and above. The following instructions may be provided and demonstrated in clinic. After the bedtime routine is complete and lights go off, the parent will come and check on the child in the following intervals: 30 sec, 1 min, 2 min, 4 min, 8 min, 16 min, etc. There is no talking after lights out except for the parent to say when he/she will be back to check again. The parent will give the child a "thumbs up" signal upon return to the room, and the child will also acknowledge the parent's presence with a return "thumbs up" signal. The parent will consistently come back at the interval indicated. This technique keeps the child in the room as it is the parent coming to check on the child which reassures the child, redirects thoughts, and helps the child fall asleep faster. After about 1 week, the time intervals can be lengthened.

Graduated extinction can be coupled with bedtime passes. At the time of lights out, the parent gives the child two bedtime passes. These can be small foamy cut-out crafts or simple index cards the child has decorated. The child is instructed that once lights go off, if they come out of the bedroom for any reason, to talk, get a drink, go to the bathroom, etc., they will have to give in a pass. In the morning, each pass that the child retains can be traded for a prize, such as 5 min of extra TV time, snacks, or other agreed upon daily incentive.

Psychophysiological insomnia

Preadolescents and adolescents may develop psychophysiological insomnia similar to adults. A polysomnogram is not required for diagnosis but should be considered if there is suspicion for co-morbid sleep disorders, such as obstructive sleep apnea.

After a thorough screen for other causes of insomnia, such as restless legs syndrome and delayed sleep phase syndrome, treatment should include age-appropriate CBT-I. This may include 4–6 visits over several weeks with a behavioral sleep medicine specialist or trained psychologist. Focus includes stimulus control, relaxation techniques, bedtime fading (gentle sleep restriction), cognitive reframing, and sleep hygiene. The main difference in treatment between children and adults with psychophysiological insomnia is that the techniques must all be modified for age-appropriate discussions with children.

Sleep maintenance insomnia

Sleep maintenance insomnia refers to multiple awakenings at night, and may include prolonged time to return to sleep. The most frequently encountered medical causes of sleep maintenance insomnia in the child include nightmare disorder and obstructive sleep apnea. Behavioral insomnia of both types mentioned above may also cause sleep maintenance insomnia.

Nightmare disorder

Nearly every child can recall a previous nightmare. Nightmare disorder occurs when the child has nighttime or daytime dysfunction as a result of repetitive "scary" dreams. A polysomnogram is not required for the diagnosis but should be performed if there is suspicion for co-morbid sleep disorders, such as obstructive sleep apnea.

Nightmares are considered to be a rapid eye movement (REM) sleep phenomenon, from which the child arouses from sleep. In most cases, nightmares have no known underlying cause but in some cases, restless legs syndrome or obstructive sleep apnea may cause arousals from REM sleep periods. Posttraumatic stress disorder, adjustment disorder or anxiety may also be related to nightmares, and these children may need additional counseling by trained specialists.

Treatment for nightmare disorder includes the removal of all daytime violence exposure. Commonly overlooked exposures include the evening news, violent video/tablet/phone games, drama-mystery shows, and "scary" movies. Nightmares may rapidly improve with changing content to non-violent sports or other non-violent entertainment.

Imagery rehearsal is another treatment option for nightmare disorder. The parent and child discuss reasonable alternative endings to the recurrent "scary" dreams. Appropriate endings should be solicited from the child and modified as needed by the parent. Additionally, the child and parent can discuss "good" things to dream about. Discussion occurs when the child is in bed, for the last 5–15 minutes before lights out, repeated nightly for at least 4 weeks. Further evaluation and treatment with a psychologist may be necessary if there are concurrent mood or anxiety disorders.

Breathing disorders

Obstructive sleep apnea (OSA)

Nighttime symptoms of obstructive sleep apnea in children include snoring, mouth breathing, gasping, choking, awakenings, enuresis, nocturia, and restlessness. Daytime symptoms include headaches, irritability, moodiness, difficulty focusing on tasks, and excessive daytime sleepiness. Of note, sleepiness in children often presents as hyperactivity. The child becomes so overly tired that he or she frequently changes activities in an attempt to stay awake. Additionally, children may do poorly in school. In one study, children performing at the lowest percentile were performing at average or above average 1 year later after treatment with adenotonsillectomy for OSA diagnosed by polysomnogram. There is also an overlap of symptoms of attention deficit hyperactivity disorder (ADHD) and obstructive sleep apnea. For example, another study showed that children diagnosed with ADHD and OSA had improvement or resolution of ADHD symptoms after treatment with adenotonsillectomy for the sleep-disordered breathing.

An overnight in-laboratory polysomnogram remains the gold standard for diagnosis of OSA in children. First-line treatment for OSA in normal weight, overweight, and obese children is adenotonsillectomy. Follow-up in sleep clinic is generally recommended approximately 12 weeks later to assess for residual symptoms and determine if a repeat polysomnogram is indicated.

In children with residual symptomatic obstructive sleep apnea despite adenotonsillectomy, oxygen or continuous positive airway pressure (CPAP) treatment may be indicated based on age and severity of sleep-disordered breathing. The FDA approves most CPAP devices for children over the age of 7 years and greater than 40 pounds (an exception is the Trilogy ventilator which can deliver CPAP to infants). However, case reports and case series show that outpatient CPAP therapy has been used safely down to age 2 years. The risks, benefits, and cleaning procedures must be explained for the child and parents to understand. The child and parent must be in favor of and agree with PAP therapy, as motivation from both parties is essential to the success of the child's treatment. Motivational interviewing techniques may be helpful to assess the willingness of the family to try CPAP therapy for an initial 4–12-week period.

For many children, the sequence of events includes polysomnogram for diagnosis of OSA, adenotonsillectomy, sustained or reoccurrence of nighttime or daytime symptoms, repeat diagnostic polysomnogram with the finding of residual OSA, and finally a CPAP titration polysomnogram. The CPAP is then ordered through a local durable medical equipment supplier.

Weight loss is recommended as adjunct therapy in any overweight child; weight loss is not recommended as sole therapy. Further considerations for treatment include saline nasal spray, steroid nasal sprays, and montelukast (Singulair). Montelukast decreases inflammatory tissues such as adenoid and tonsillar tissue to increase airflow. For children too young for or who do not tolerate CPAP, supplemental oxygen may improve hypoxia. Supplemental oxygen does not treat obstructive sleep apnea. It is recommended to observe carbon dioxide values during a trial of supplemental oxygen to ensure that its application does not induce hypercapnia.

Orthodontic treatment may be an option for children with very high-arched hard palates, as rapid palate expansion has shown promising results in treating pediatric OSA. Depending on the age of the child, if jaw growth is complete, an oral appliance may also improve or resolve OSA.

Positional therapy can be attempted if a particular position is associated with a significant reduction in the OSA severity. Parents should exercise caution in elevating the head of the bed in children as children often end up at the bottom of the mattress. Specialty pillows or belts may be purchased online or from medical equipment suppliers.

As newer therapy options emerge for adults, these will require testing for effectiveness and safety in children. For example, Provent, a nightly-use nasal device with a one-way valve, held in place by a hypoallergenic adhesive, was recently approved by the FDA for the treatment of OSA in adults. Its effectiveness and safety have not yet been tested in children.

Lastly, children with special considerations such as craniofacial dysmorphology may require additional surgical interventions performed by otolaryngology, oral-maxillofacial or plastic surgeons.

Other breathing disorders

It is difficult to differentiate obstructive sleep apnea, central sleep apnea, and hypercapnia by clinical history; the in-laboratory polysomnogram clarifies the diagnosis. If central sleep apnea is observed with a Central Apnea Index >4, further work-up may be necessary, including evaluation with detailed neurological examination and magnetic resonance imaging of the brain and cardiac evaluation with electrocardiogram and echocardiogram. Hypercapnia may accompany OSA and treatment is often similar to that for OSA though in specific cases, more aggressive ventilation may need to be considered.

An additional respiratory sleep disorder is congenital central hypoventilation syndrome (CCHS), also known as Ondine's curse. Often this disorder is diagnosed during the neonatal period due to respiratory difficulty and failure to thrive. Many children die undiagnosed or the death may be misdiagnosed as SIDS. In this disorder, the child hypoventilates and central respiratory centers do not respond correctly to the hypercapnia. A polysomnogram is required to diagnose this disorder; occasionally the key features of CCHS on a polysomnogram are the first clues to the diagnosis. In stage N3, the child will be relatively hypoxic compared to other stages of sleep. Furthermore, on the sleep study, the carbon dioxide values (CO_2) will begin to rise without adequate respiratory compensation. Evaluation includes checking for a Phox2B gene mutation, of which several have been identified specific to this disorder. Treatment includes pulmonary collaboration with the child, often requiring mechanical ventilation at night for appropriate respiration.

Hypersomnias

This group of disorders includes narcolepsy with and without cataplexy, idiopathic hypersomnia, and recurrent hypersomnias such as Klein–Levin and menstrual-related hypersomnia. Narcolepsy has a peak incidence at 15 years of age in children. Although the incidence is 1 per 2000, narcolepsy may be difficult to diagnose because of poor sleep hygiene and the irregular sleep schedules of many teenagers. Additionally, hypersomnia disorders should be considered in children if they require naps after previously giving them up, or parents are requested to remove the child from school or hold back a school grade due to sleepiness. Subjective testing with a pediatric-modified Epworth Sleepiness Scale may be helpful; a Multiple Sleep Latency Test (MSLT) should be considered for children who score >13, and performed on the day following the in-laboratory overnight polysomnogram.

The diagnosis of narcolepsy requires daily excessive sleepiness for 3 months. Additional features

Table 15.4 Normal values for the MSLT in children

Tanner stage	Mean sleep latency (min)	Standard deviation (min)
Stage 1	19.0	1.6
Stage 2	18.5	1.9
Stage 3	16.1	3.8
Stage 4	15.8	3.4
Stage 5	16.6	2.1

Adapted from Hoban TF, Chervin RD. Assessment of sleepiness in children. *Semin Pediatr Neurol* 2001; **8**(4): 216–28.

may include cataplexy, hypnogogic hallucinations, sleep paralysis, and fragmented overnight sleep. If a child/parent replies affirmatively when asked if the child feels weak with strong emotion, it is helpful to ask them to describe the exact details of the episode.

Cataplexy is differentiated from syncope as the child maintains consciousness and can hear and see surroundings. The child is only able to use extraocular and respiratory muscles. Examples of cataplexy include bilateral facial drooping or loss of expression, neck bobbling, knee bobbling or, in extreme cases, falling to the ground. Children may have difficulty describing the cataplexy due to a limited vocabulary or ability to describe the sensation. Furthermore, strong emotions in children may differ from adults such as when the child is being disciplined or during physical education class or recess. In children, cataplexy may not occur at the time of onset of severe sleepiness.

An overnight in-laboratory polysomnogram followed by a daytime MSLT is recommended for children aged 7 years and older, as younger children may still take naps and be considered physiologically normal. The overnight polysomnogram will ensure that no other sleep disorders may be accounting for the child's sleepiness. Pathologic sleep latency values are based on Tanner staging (Table 15.4). The protocol for MSLT testing can be found on the American Academy of Sleep Medicine website (www.aasmnet.org/Resources/Practice Parameters/PP_MSLTMWT.pdf). Though by protocol antidepressants or stimulant medications are typically stopped prior to this test, it may be acceptable to have parents continue the child's medications due to concerns around the child's function at school and home off their medications for the

optimal 2-week (or longer for some medications) washout period. Discontinuation or interruption of selective serotonin reuptake inhibitors (SSRIs) and stimulant medication 1–3 days before or on the day of MSLT testing can cause hypersomnia or a REM sleep-rebound phenomenon and thus false-positive results.

Sleep onset REM periods (SOREMP) on the MSLT (seen typically in adults with narcolepsy) may take up to 3 years to develop from time of symptom onset in children. Thus serial testing can be considered, but is not required if the child and parent provide a clear classic description of cataplexy. A "temporary" diagnosis of idiopathic hypersomnia may be appropriate if the child does not have cataplexy, does not have at least two SOREMPs between the overnight sleep study and daytime MSLT, and yet has an abnormally short sleep latency on the MSLT.

A few unique features of childhood narcolepsy exist. Naps may be longer and non-refreshing. Treatment options include behavior and lifestyle modifications. It is recommended that children increase daytime exercise and activity and avoid situations which may precipitate cataplexy. Traditional stimulants to treat daytime sleepiness are used at the same doses as for other disorders such as ADHD. Cataplexy may also improve with use of traditional stimulants. For resistant cataplexy, very low-dose selective norepinephrine serotonin reuptake inhibitors (such as 37.5 mg venlafaxine daily) or other selective serotonin reuptake inhibitors or tricyclic antidepressants may provide relief. Case reports and series have also discussed use of sodium hydroxybuterate (Xyrem), modafanil (Provigil), and armodafanil (Nuvigil) in children with narcolepsy, as these are FDA approved for use in narcolepsy in adults.

✋ CAUTION

Cataplexy safety
A discussion on safety at every visit should review avoidance of heights or monkey-bars on playgrounds, swimming, cooking, driving, and other activities during which having cataplexy or sleep attacks could be dangerous. Some activities may be reasonable with close adult supervision.

If narcolepsy is suspected in a young child (preschool or earlier), consider magnetic resonance imaging (MRI) to evaluate for central nervous system lesions that may be responsible for the excessive sleepiness.

Circadian rhythm disturbances

See above discussion of delayed sleep phase type. Other forms of circadian dysfunction are less common in children.

Parasomnias

Parasomnias refer to unusual motor activity during sleep and can be divided into non-rapid eye movement (NREM) and REM sleep parasomnias. NREM sleep parasomnias include sleep terrors, sleepwalking, sleep talking, confusional arousals, and enuresis. REM sleep parasomnias include nightmares, as described above, and, very rarely in children, REM sleep behavior disorder. Additionally, sleep-related seizures may mimic parasomnias; more information is included in the section below.

Non-rapid eye movement sleep parasomnias occur when a partial arousal occurs during NREM sleep, most commonly stage N3 sleep (also known as slow-wave sleep). The most commonly observed triggers in children include a poor sleep environment, sleep deprivation, RLS, and OSA. If persistent parasomnias occur despite treatment with a quiet, dark appropriate sleep space, with adequate time in bed and treatment for RLS or other known sleep disorders, then scheduled awakenings may be instituted or, if absolutely necessary, off-label use of medication such as a benzodiazepine can be considered. A scheduled awakening is performed approximately 30 min prior to the typical time when the episodes occur; the parent gently awakens the child just enough to open their eyes, then the child is allowed to fall back to sleep immediately.

For children who sleepwalk, it is paramount to ensure safety.

> ✋ CAUTION
>
> **Sleepwalking safety**
> Parents are encouraged to purchase door alarms ($8–15) from home improvement stores; these alarms can be placed on any doors or windows that exit the home. In addition, furniture with sharp corners and edges should be padded or removed.

Dangerous items such as keys to cars, knives, and guns should be kept locked at night. Furthermore, children should avoid sleeping on the top bunk of bunk beds. Children may reduce harm by sleeping on the floor and/or on the ground floor of the home.

Nocturnal epileptic events

It can be difficult to differentiate a parasomnia such as a night terror from an epileptic paroxysmal event during sleep by the parent's description alone. Clues suggestive of epileptic events include stereotypical movements night after night, eye blinking, head turning to one side, limb posturing, rhythmic movements, drooling, or tongue biting; the event occurs from stage N1 or N2 sleep, and similar episodes have occurred when the child is awake. Clues suggestive of parasomnias include occurrence 1–2 hours (or longer) after the child has fallen asleep, or event occurs from stage N3. During sleep terrors, the child may appear frightened. Some clinical features are present in both epileptic events and parasomnias: occurrence multiple times per night, confusion after the event, and amnesia for the events. Videos recorded by parents and extended EEG, such as 24–48-hours monitoring or polysomnography with full EEG montage, are often helpful in distinguishing the disorders.

Nocturnal epilepsy syndromes
(by typical age of onset)

- *Infantile spasms*: age of onset from birth to 18 months of age. Parents may note morning body spasms. EEG shows hypsarrhythmia, high-amplitude, irregular epileptiform discharges. Of note, benign myoclonus of infancy is a disorder in which the infant appears to be having seizures, with rhythmic myoclonic jerks during drowsiness or sleep. However, these are not epileptic events. Benign myoclonus of infancy is a disorder of NREM sleep which can occur between birth and age 3 years, with normal sleep EEG. Furthermore, awakening the child resolves all rhythmic motor activity in benign myoclonus of infancy.
- *Benign epilepsy of childhood with occipital paroxysms*: typically presents between ages 2 and 6 years, with parents noting eye deviation, with

autonomic instability of heart rate, respirations, and blood pressure. Sleep EEG shows epileptiform discharges over the occipital regions.

- *Benign epilepsy with centrotemporal spikes*: age of onset 3–13 years; this is the most common partial epilepsy syndrome in children. Parents may describe the child having twitches of the lower face, lips, and around the mouth, drooling, and dysarthria. Sleep EEG shows spikes in the central and temporal regions.
- *Landau–Kleffner syndrome*: typically presents between ages 4 to 6 years, with language regression and nocturnal episodes.
- *Frontal lobe epilepsy and paroxysmal nocturnal dystonia*: mean age of onset is 14 years; events can range from brief sudden arousals to minutes of ambulation; nocturnal behaviors and motor activity may be simple to complex and include aggressive outbursts. Autosomal dominant nocturnal frontal lobe epilepsy has been described; family history may help with diagnosis.
- *Juvenile myoclonic epilepsy*: presents typically during teenage years; seizure activity typically occurs upon awakening in the mornings, and can sometimes be subtle and mistaken for staring spells or clumsiness. Family history may help with diagnosis. Avoidance of sleep deprivation and alcohol is recommended.
- *Electrical status epilepticus in slow-wave sleep*: also has been described in childhood, with continuous spike and wave discharges during stage N3; no epileptiform discharges are observed in REM sleep.

Summary

It is recommended that children with epilepsy be queried about sleep symptoms as sleep disorders may further worsen their seizure frequency and duration. Several small studies show that treatment of obstructive sleep apnea may decrease seizure frequency.

Sleep-related movements

This category includes RLS, periodic limb movement disorder (PLMD) and sleep-related rhythmic movements such as body rocking, head banging, and humming. RLS has been described in detail above.

Periodic limb movements of sleep are a polysomnographic finding that may not cause symptoms.

Conversely, RLS is a sensation or urge to move the legs or affected limbs during wake. The definition of a periodic limb movement (PLM) series on a sleep study includes at least four leg movements (increase in electromyographic voltage over the baseline muscle tone) in a defined time period of at least 5 sec apart and no more than 90 sec apart. A PLM index of five limb movements or more per hour of sleep is abnormal in children. Periodic limb movement disorder should be diagnosed if there are >5 PLMs per hour on the sleep study, no RLS symptoms, and the child has daytime dysfunction. The suspected pathological pathway and treatment are the same as for RLS.

Head banging, body rocking, humming, and additional variations of rhythmic movements typically occur at the onset of sleep. Thus, they may occur only as the child is laying down to sleep, or may continue intermittently throughout the night based on the child's normal, expected arousals and awakenings. Sleep-related movements should not be considered a disorder unless there is resultant daytime dysfunction.

Treatment of an underlying sleep-fragmenting disorder such as RLS or OSA will decrease the opportunity for cortical arousals. This will in turn decrease the occurrence of the sleep-related movements. For example, iron or other treatment for restless legs syndrome will help to lessen the leg pains, consolidate sleep, and decrease the frequency of arousals and awakenings, thereby decreasing the child's need for body rocking to self-soothe back to sleep. Similarly, with resolution of breathing disturbance in children who undergo treatment for OSA, sleep becomes more consolidated with less opportunity for sleep-related rhythmic movements. Parents should also be reassured that sleep-related movements generally lessen over time and are most commonly benign without known long-term medical or behavioral effects.

Conclusion

This chapter has reviewed several pediatric sleep symptoms and disorders commonly seen in pediatric neurology clinics. Neurological disorders may be exacerbated by sleep disturbances in children. Thorough sleep history taking and treatment of sleep disorders may yield higher success rates for the concomitant treatment of neurological disorders.

Further reading

Aurora RN, Lamm CI, Zak RS, et al. Practice parameters for the non-respiratory indications for polysomnography and multiple sleep latency testing for children. *Sleep* 2012; **35**(11): 1467–73.

Aurora RN, Zak RS, Karippot A, et al. Practice parameters for the respiratory indications for polysomnography in children. *Sleep* 2011; **34**(3): 379–88.

Hoban TF. Sleep disorders in children. *Ann N Y Acad Sci* 2010; **1184**: 1–14.

Marcus CL, Brooks LJ, Ward SD, et al. Diagnosis and management of childhood obstructive sleep apnea syndrome. *Pediatrics* 2012; **130**: e714–e755.

Morgenthaler TI, Owens J, Alessi C, et al. Practice parameters for behavioral treatment of bedtime problems and night wakings in infants and young children. *Sleep* 2006; **29**(10): 1277–81.

Standards of Practice Committee of the American Academy of Sleep Medicine. Practice parameters for clinical use of the multiple sleep latency test and the maintenance of wakefulness test. *Sleep* 2005; **28**(1): 113–21.

Vendrame M, Kothare SV. Epileptic and nonepileptic events out of sleep in children. *J Clin Neurophysiol* 2011; **28**: 111–19.

Wise MS, Arand DL, Auger RR, Brooks SN, Watson NF. Treatment of narcolepsy and other hypersomnias of central origin. *Sleep* 2007; **30**(12): 1712–27.

Index

Note: Page references in *italics* refer to Figures; those in **bold** refer to Tables and Boxes

Sleep Medicine in Neurology, First Edition. Edited by Douglas B. Kirsch.
© 2014 John Wiley & Sons, Ltd. Published 2014 by John Wiley & Sons, Ltd.